THE INFORMED PATIENT

A volume in the series

THE CULTURE AND POLITICS OF HEALTH CARE WORK
edited by Suzanne Gordon and Sioban Nelson

A list of titles in this series is available at cornellpress.cornell.edu.

THE INFORMED PATIENT

A COMPLETE GUIDE TO A HOSPITAL STAY

Karen A. Friedman, MD, and Sara L. Merwin, MPH

ILR Press
an imprint of
Cornell University Press
Ithaca and London

First published 2017 by Cornell University Press
Printed in the United States of America

Library of Congress Cataloging-in-Publication Data

Names: Friedman, Karen A., author. | Merwin, Sara L., author.
Title: The informed patient : a complete guide to a hospital stay / Karen A.
    Friedman, MD, and Sara L. Merwin, MPH.
Description: Ithaca : ILR Press, an imprint of Cornell University Press, 2017. |
    Series: The culture and politics of health care work | Includes index.
Identifiers: LCCN 2017016231 (print) | LCCN 2017017264 (ebook) |
    ISBN 9781501714061 (pdf) | ISBN 9781501714078 (epub/mobi) |
    ISBN 9781501709951 (pbk. : alk. paper)
Subjects: LCSH: Hospital patients—Popular works. | Hospital care—Popular
    works. | Patient education—Popular works. | Patient advocacy—Popular
    works. | Consumer education—Popular works.
Classification: LCC RA965.6 (ebook) | LCC RA965.6 .F75 2017 (print) |
    DDC 362.11—dc23
LC record available at https://lccn.loc.gov/2017016231

This book contains information that is intended to help the readers be better informed consumers of health care. It is presented as general advice on health care. Always consult your doctor for your individual needs.

Contents

How It All Began and Why We Wrote This Book

It began with a shared office—five internist physicians and a research coordinator sharing a small space in a highly regarded suburban New York hospital. It was an atmosphere ripe for the exchange of ideas. Karen (the doctor) and Sara (the researcher) soon became fast friends, the work in the hospital the common denominator. Karen took care of patients and trained young doctors, while Sara interacted with research subjects and the doctors and nurses who took care of them. We talked about the patients' illnesses, we discussed the perils of being hospitalized, and when Sara needed advice about how to help her family members and friends get good medical treatment, Karen and the hospital-based internists were right there to answer questions.

An idea was about to be born.

Wouldn't it be great to give the average person—who didn't have access to this kind of advice—the inside scoop on what to expect during a hospital stay?

Wouldn't it be ideal to create an inpatient reference book with all kinds of information, not just medical but practical as well?

Wouldn't it be wonderful to give patients in the hospital insights about how to ask the right questions to protect themselves and to get better care?

We were thus inspired to write a book to take some of the mystery and confusion out of the hospital experience. The book opens the door and allows the reader an entry into the world of the hospital.

And so this collaboration was started. We talked, we outlined, we wrote. The months went by (actually years). Karen got promoted, and

Sara changed departments. Still, we talked, we added details, we wrote. Sara's mother got sick; advocacy skills were urgently needed. This book waited. Eventually it got reborn. (Sara's mother got better.)

The following stories illustrate how different people dealt with their hospital stays in different ways.

A married couple that we know are both young, highly successful lawyers. They are at the top of their fields and often quoted in the media. A few years ago, the husband became quite ill after a routine office procedure. His symptoms worsened, he was unable to work or eat, and after several days it was determined that he needed to be admitted to the hospital to receive IV antibiotics. It turned out that he had a serious infection, an unusual but not completely unexpected result of certain kinds of biopsies. After a long and miserable day and a half in the emergency room waiting for a bed, he was finally admitted to a room. By this point he was not getting better, and he was extremely uncomfortable with pain, nausea, and fevers. When we visited him in his hospital room, we saw the state he was in. This previously strong and healthy person was suffering and unable to do anything about it—or even to ask for pain relief. He did not question whether his doctors and nurses were taking the best possible care of him. To our shock, his wife, an empowered, extroverted attorney—who in the service of her clients advocates magnificently—seemed resigned and complacent. She was unable to do so much as ask the nurse for antinausea medication, let alone request a consultation with an infectious disease specialist to see why her husband was not getting better. This is an example of the mental paralysis that often sets in when we find ourselves confronted with the unfamiliar world of the hospital.

The second story is about Sara's youngest son. Harry, at age thirteen, was diagnosed with ulcerative colitis, an inflammatory disease, which causes pain and diarrhea. The oral medications prescribed for him seemed to have no effect, and, a small child to begin with, he continued to lose weight and have high fevers and was unable to go to school, eat normally, or play. His excellent pediatric gastroenterologist sensibly wanted to keep him out of the hospital but advised us that we would know when we would have to bring him to the emergency room if it got too bad. Sure enough, that night arrived, and Harry was brought to the emergency room of the local children's hospital, thin, debilitated, and barely able to walk. He spent the next eight days, including Hanukkah and Christmas, in the hospital getting intravenous fluids and medications. Here is where the surprising part comes in. Without any tutoring from his mother, Sara, who works in a large hospital system, every single time a nurse brought his medications Harry asked to see what bag of medication he or she was giving him. Every time a nurse finished giving him new IV medications, he asked if the intravenous lines had been flushed. At one point, when a pediatric resident asked Harry if he wanted ibuprofen for his pain, he told the doctor in training, "I can't have ibuprofen because I have ulcerative colitis." In addition to advocating for himself effectively, he displayed consideration for the hospital staff around him. He thanked each and every person who came into his room—not only the doctors and nurses but also the woman who brought the lunch tray and the man who emptied the trash. His assertiveness and his preparedness served him well.

This book reflects so much of what we have learned from our experiences with patients, with research subjects, with family and friends. We are excited to share what we know with you, with your caregivers, and, we hope, with your health care providers.

ACKNOWLEDGMENTS

There are many people we would like to thank for helping to make this book happen. Suzanne Gordon, our editor, believed in us from the start. We can never thank her enough for her time, commitment, and support. Frances Benson, our publisher at Cornell University Press, gave us the encouragement and praise we needed through the process.

Thank you, Deb Chasman, for pointing us in the right direction; we are forever grateful.

We thank our hands-on helpers: Alan Fein, MD, intensivist extraordinaire, who guided us about ICUs; Paul Levin, MD, who helped us find the "person" in surgical patients and provided technical advice; Lorie Greenberg, MD, who informed our comments on pediatric patients; Rocio Crabb, who organized us; Matt Rothschild, who made our sentences make sense; Ross Lumpkin, the sensational glossarist. Thanks to David Rosenberg, MD, MPH, for seating us next to each other in that famous office and for telling us we should not give up on the book.

Support comes in many forms. We have had many good listeners in our friends and families. Ted Merwin supplied practical advice gleaned from his own experience. Our husbands and children cheered us on and were endlessly patient about the hours we took to accomplish this writing. Other friends and family members provided material for the vignettes and gave permission to tell their stories.

Finally we thank our team members: our professional colleagues, our teachers, our residents, and of course, the patients. We learn from you every day.

THE INFORMED PATIENT

CHAPTER 1

Why You Need This Book and How to Use This Book

Why do you need this book? Honestly, it's because everyone ends up in a hospital sooner or later and very few of us have the knowledge, skills, and confidence to ensure the best possible care.

We have written this book in response to our observation that most individuals do not come into the hospital well prepared with either advocacy skills or an advocate to help them navigate an inpatient stay during this emotional time. Health care has become ever more complex with increased technology in the age of information. Health care providers are busier than ever before and are also inundated with changing technology, rapidly advancing treatments, and a heightened paperwork burden. As a consequence, more vigilance by the patient is required to remain safe.

SOME STATISTICS

Here are a few figures about hospital stays that may surprise or alarm you:

- There are 34.4 million hospital discharges per year in the United States alone, not even including the Veterans Health Administration system.
- The average length of stay for hospital visits is 4.8 days.
- Between 210,000 and 400,000 patient deaths a year may be attributed to preventable medical errors in U.S. hospitals.
- Ninety-nine thousand patients die as a result of hospital-acquired infections each year, according to the Agency for Healthcare, Research and Quality.

MEDICAL ERRORS AND BEYOND

Patient safety has become a major concern of the general public; policy-makers; and local, state, and national government. Frequent news coverage has been devoted to individuals who were victims of serious medical errors. In 1999, the Institute of Medicine published a book called *To Err Is Human*. This was a groundbreaking report because it exposed just how dangerous a hospital stay can be. It opened our eyes to the real risks of a hospital stay, asserting that ninety-nine thousand patients die every year from preventable medical errors, an estimate that has risen dramatically since 1999. When we talk about medical errors, we mean two different kinds. The first is an *error of commission*—a fancy way of saying that something specifically incorrect was done or given to a patient. An *error of omission*, on the other hand, means that the patient did not get the medication or procedure or provision of care necessary, or that something varied from what the medical profession calls the *standard of care*.

In its 2003 follow-up report, *Patient Safety: Achieving a New Standard of Care*, the Institute of Medicine emphasized the importance of standardizing and better managing information on patient safety to reduce the risk of harm and ensure good care.

A study in the journal *Health Affairs* showed that one-third of hospital patients have *adverse events* (unwanted and potential problems resulting from medical care), and approximately 7 percent are harmed permanently or die as a result. This study brought new attention to the safety issues that were originally brought to the forefront by the two Institute of Medicine books. Unfortunately, even though hospitals are making headway in the arena of patient safety, it is still unsafe to be hospitalized and will continue to be so.

WHY YOU NEED TO BE AN ADVOCATE
OR HAVE AN ADVOCATE

Medicine as it is practiced now is so complex and time is so limited to health care providers that certain aspects of care in the hospital can be overlooked or mistaken. We want to make sure that things go as smoothly as possible by helping you become well informed and encouraging you to speak up when you have concerns.

Advocating for yourself or your loved ones in the hospital is not easy. Even if hospitals were perfectly run, immaculately clean, and staffed uniformly with kind and generous human beings, it would still be daunting and bewildering to be an inpatient. And this is because when we are ill or fear for our loved ones, we are emotionally vulnerable. This is true even for those of us who work in health care.

It is vitally important to be assertive (NOT aggressive). So many of us have learned to be unnecessarily deferential to doctors; this is particularly true of the older generation, whose members would not think of questioning the doctor. Times have changed. It is a mistake to blindly accept treatment or submit to tests recommended by your health providers; it is perfectly reasonable to ask questions and to be a participant in your own care. In fact, "shared decision making" is a concept that has been embraced by the medical community, and it relies on patients to be actively involved in their health care and to make decisions in concert with their health care providers. Increasingly, there is an emphasis on patient preferences and values to help medical professionals make the right choices suited to the specific needs of the individuals they care for.

The cornerstone of this book is that you, the patient, can become an active participant in your own health care story. Recently and fortunately, the medical field has moved away from a paternalistic approach that put physicians at the top of the hierarchy and you, the patient, at the bottom; you were expected to follow directions without questioning the doctor's reasons and rationale. When it comes to choosing between treatment options, it is important for you to express your own wishes.

We want you to have the best possible outcome from a hospital stay; all patients have the right to insist that the health care providers and hospital staff do the very best by them.

WHAT YOU WILL LEARN

We are going to give you a great deal of information about what happens in the hospital: how modern hospitals are organized, the roles and descriptions of the various professionals and other hospital staff taking care of you, what tests you might encounter, common medications, how you can get help when you need it, and what you can expect during your stay.

HERE IS HOW YOU CAN USE THIS BOOK TO BEST ADVANTAGE

Think of this book as a necessary training manual. If you have a planned surgery or have elderly or ill family members, you will certainly have to deal with a hospital visit. Given the complex nature of hospital care, you will need to educate yourself in order to be prepared. This book is intended to be a valuable resource to help you navigate the turbulent waters of hospital issues and problems. Managing the hospital experience for yourself or your loved one is your new job. Now you will begin training so that you will be prepared and ultimately successful.

You can pick and choose topics according to your need. You do not have to read this book in the order in which it is written or in its entirety. You can start anywhere, depending on what your specific need is. What you will find is a kind of reference book, filled with details and information. However, there are certain ideas and principles that we feel are so intrinsic to your success as an advocate that we have highlighted them as tips and stressed them for emphasis.

Tips

We have emphasized and repeated certain elements that may seem obvious but that in the setting of caring for yourself or a hospitalized loved one you may forget. You will see these tips interspersed throughout the text. They are to remind you about your role in helping yourself or your family member.

Sidebars

When we want to delve a little more deeply into a topic, we present sidebars. Usually this is a more detailed explanation of something discussed in the section adjacent to the sidebar. Or it might be an insight about hospital workings not typically known to the general public.

Vignettes

Of course it is not possible to describe all the conceivable situations patients and their families will experience during an inpatient stay. We have chosen some typical types of scenarios to paint a picture of the universal questions and qualms that you might have. When appropriate, at the end of the clinical vignette, we propose a solution to a commonly encountered problem.

ABOUT TERMINOLOGY

The "Patient" and the "Doctor"

Throughout this book you will see us refer to "the patient," as "yourself," "your family member," or "your loved one." That person could be you, a spouse, a child, a parent or other relative, a friend, or a neighbor. In certain instances, a patient will be able to advocate on his or her own. More often than not, because of fear, pain, or confusion, patients find themselves at a loss to assert themselves when hospitalized. For convenience, we will use the terms "you," "your patient," "the patient," and even "your loved one" to mean the person for whom something needs to be done.

Likewise, we will alternate between using the terms "doctor,"

> **Vocabulary and Alphabet Soup**
>
> Not only is the world of medicine confusing and hard for the layperson to understand, but it has its own language, made up of Latin and scientific terms. To deal with all this vocabulary, medical professionals and hospital workers abbreviate like crazy. And here's a little secret: very often the abbreviations used by one specialty mean something completely different for another specialty. For example, ARF could mean acute renal (kidney) failure or acute respiratory (breathing) failure. Understanding some basic terms and abbreviations can help you navigate the hospital stay. You will see these terms in italics, often with an explanation afterward in parentheses. And there is a handy glossary at the end of this book.

"physician," "health care team," and "health care provider" to mean the licensed individuals who are responsible for your care. Some of them may be medical doctors (MDs), doctors of osteopathy (DOs), nurse practitioners (NPs), nurses (RNs), or physician assistants (PAs). When we refer to "health care professionals," we include social workers, respiratory therapists, and physical therapists in addition to the providers mentioned above.

Vocabulary and Terms

In the medical world, some words that we are familiar with in everyday life take on a particular meaning. You will hear certain words over and over again: "assess," "evaluate," "manage," "follow," "indication," "attending." It may be difficult to make sense of what you are hearing, particularly at first. Further, there is a medical lexicon unto itself filled with Latin and scientific words, and it will be impossible to understand all the medical talk around you. We have italicized many terms, explained their meaning inside the world of the hospital, and put them in a glossary at the end of the book for easy reference.

TIP   Take Notes

Take notes: Write everything down!!! We cannot emphasize this advice enough. Use the pages in the book if you wish or carry a notepad. No one can integrate medical information during a serious illness or trauma, and no one expects you to remember what the doctor says. We strongly suggest that you compile questions to pose to your health care providers and that you write down the information they give you to help you understand what it is happening and when it will happen.

CHAPTER 2

The Changing Landscape of Medicine

Almost everything about how medicine is practiced in the United States and the developed world has changed over the past twenty years: there has been a proliferation of new tests, new technology, new medications, and new specialties. Thanks to these improvements, along with better nutrition and preventive care, the population is living longer. Along with this extension in life expectancy come more medical problems. It is impossible for doctors, much less laypersons, to keep up with all these changes. More difficult still, in the new paradigm the patient is the consumer. To be an uninformed consumer when it comes to health care puts you at a distinct disadvantage.

We are all bombarded with print, TV, radio, and Internet advertisements for medications, doctors' practices, medical technologies, specialized procedures, and even specific hospitals. Everyone is selling wares in the medical marketplace. And everyone wants your business. Health care is very, very big business. It didn't use to be this way. Your doctor knew what medications you needed and you followed **his** (emphasis intentional) advice. You didn't question, and you didn't think about other options or choices. You didn't have to "prepare" for a doctor's visit or trip to the hospital by reading up. You didn't have to research which medications would be best for you. In short, you were not a partner in your health care, nor were you an informed consumer. But much has changed, and nowhere are the changes more evident than in the hospital. Most patients are diagnosed by laboratory results and imaging techniques. Physical diagnosis is a dying art. Decisions about patient care may be made in a room far away from the patient instead of at the bedside.

MORE CHANGES: HOSPITALISTS VERSUS GPs AND FAMILY DOCTORS WHO COME TO THE HOSPITAL

Among the biggest changes in medicine is that more and more often, there are doctors who work ONLY in the hospital and do not see patients on the outside. These doctors are called *hospitalists.* This movement has mostly been in general internal medicine (practitioners we used to call GPs, general practitioners, or family doctors), but it has been so successful that now there are pediatric and neurology hospitalists, as well as hospitalists *managing* (taking care of) medical issues for surgical patients. This is a trend that is here to

Primary Care Provider (PCP) Can Be Any One of the Following:

General practitioner—that is, an internist, either MD (medical doctor) or DO (doctor of osteopathy); family practitioner (FP); nurse practitioner (NP); or physician assistant (PA)

Specialist Can Be in Any of the Subspecialties of Internal Medicine:

Allergy and immunology, cardiovascular disease, critical care medicine, endocrinology, diabetes and metabolism, gastroenterology, geriatrics, hematology, hospice and palliative medicine, infectious disease, nephrology, oncology, pulmonary disease, rheumatology, and sleep medicine

stay. It has proven to be efficient and been demonstrated to improve care, although it may seem more than a little impersonal to patients and their families.

What this means is that the doctor, *generalist* or *specialist,* you see for office visits may not be seeing you in the hospital at all, or if so, less frequently. Even if a hospitalist does not take care of you, the likelihood is that if you see a doctor in a large group, the junior physician of the group, even if he or she is not your own doctor, will be looking in on you in the hospital.

RAPPORT AND COMFORT VERSUS EFFICIENCY AND QUALITY CARE

Although the reliance on hospitalists may seem impersonal to you, it does allow your *primary care provider (PCP)* or general practitioner to give you more attention when you are seen in the office. In addition, it turns out that there really is quite a difference between the doctoring skills needed in the hospital and those needed in the office or clinic. There is now so much to learn in medicine that this new kind of specialization makes very good sense and ultimately saves you money by keeping health care costs down. While some internists can successfully manage both arenas, many struggle to find the right balance.

You may find it somewhat off-putting to be cared for by a complete stranger rather than your own primary care provider, someone with whom you have had a relationship for years. However, the doctors who work exclusively in the hospital are really well equipped with knowledge and training to take the best possible care of you. On an interpersonal level this may be of little comfort to you when you or your family member is ill.

The new system has proved to be better for patients and doctors alike, and you can remain confident that patient safety and well-being are enhanced by allowing certain doctors to focus all their attention on taking care of hospitalized patients.

OTHER PRIMARY CARE PROVIDERS

There has been a large growth in a new kind of health care provider to help relieve the tremendous pressure on physicians to evaluate and treat patients. Since the mid-1960s and the passage of Medicare and Medicaid legislation, there has been a chronic shortage of primary care physicians in the US health care system. Other health care providers have picked up some of the load. *Nurse practitioners (NPs), registered nurses (RNs),* and *physician assistants (PAs)* all have had specialized training to take care of patients in partnership with (and sometimes instead of) physicians. In most states, according to regulations, NPs and PAs are licensed to write prescriptions in the same manner as doctors.

Although there are many critics of these terms, nurse practitioners and physician assistants are sometimes referred to as *midlevel providers* or *physician extenders.* We present these terms for completeness, since you might hear them during your hospital stay, but we will not be using them in the remainder of the book. Nurse practitioners and physician assistants have been termed mid-levels because their training is less than that of doctors and the level of health care they are licensed to administer is different from that of RNs. They have a minimum of a bachelor's degree, and most have also completed graduate or master's-level education.

HIPAA

By this point most people have run into the HIPAA privacy law, which was put into effect in 1996. HIPAA stands for the Health Insurance Portability and Accountability Act and was signed into law by then president Bill Clinton. HIPAA was designed to protect personal medical information from getting into the wrong hands. Although this law creates extra paperwork and sometimes acts as a barrier that prevents families from obtaining information in the hospital, it does protect patients' privacy. Particularly in this age of electronic

HIPAA

Although the HIPAA rules protect patient privacy, it may be advantageous to share health information with other individuals. There are several ways in which a family member or legally authorized guardian may obtain HIPAA information about a patient. The patient who signs the HIPAA form is able to designate who else may see this information. A person can make health care decisions for another individual using a health care power of attorney. In that case, the person is considered the "personal representative." Patients who do not have cognitive capacity to take care of their own medical needs will have another individual sign on their behalf. Of course, minor children automatically assign HIPAA privilege to parents and guardians. In emergency situations, the private health information may be revealed to a family member or friend.

information, there is a need to be extra careful about a person's individual data or information. In fact, what HIPAA does is protect the security and privacy of your medical data. So the HIPAA forms are beneficial to you, and you should not hesitate to sign them.

HEALTH SYSTEMS AND HOSPITALS: THE ACUTE OR SHORT- STAY HOSPITAL AND BEYOND

How each hospital works and is organized and how it is run—its *culture*—is different, and therefore your experience will vary from hospital to hospital. Hospital culture is influenced by many factors—for example, by whether the hospital is public, private, for profit, corporate, or owned by a religious entity. Additionally, hospitals can be grouped by the level of care they provide and the degree of complexity and intensity of services. To further complicate the classification of hospitals, there has been a trend to centralize services. What this means is that while your local hospital might once have provided all types of services (*obstetrics, orthopaedics*, medical illness care, and so on), these days you might find that to conserve and concentrate services and to improve efficiency, the women's services (*obstetrics* and *gynecology*, or ob/gyn for short) have been located in one hospital while the orthopaedic (fracture repair; knee, spine, and hip surgeries, for example) have been put in another hospital. Although it may seem inconvenient to you, this concentration of expertise and specialized care almost always serves the patient more favorably.

Increasingly, you will hear hospitals called *medical centers* or even "centers." This usually denotes a hospital with many different kinds of services to offer. At the top of the heap is a *health system* or *health care system*. A health system is a group of hospitals and health care facilities (which might include rehabilitation centers, outpatient offices, and nursing homes) that is owned and managed centrally. The emergence of health systems is a huge trend and, like so many other enterprises, is driven, unsurprisingly, by economics. The simplest way to explain this is to think about buying things in bulk. Just as people will often go to a big-box store to save money, it turns out to be cheaper to purchase medical goods and services in large quantities. As a result, large and small hospitals have chosen (or been forced, in some cases) to join a health system to continue to operate at a profit.

To describe the phenomenon of health care systems and explain hospital types, we would need to write several books. Here we will instead briefly describe some hospital types so you will better understand what to expect.

Community Hospital

A *community hospital* is almost exactly what it sounds like: it is situated in your town or county and it is your local go-to place for illness and accidents. It provides a variety of services but not necessarily at the highest, or *superspecialization,* level. For routine care, the community hospital is ideal. Examples of these kinds of services are delivering a baby, setting a broken arm, treating you for pneumonia or flu requiring an inpatient stay, and even assessing your chest pain. Some people feel that the care is more personalized and less cold at the local community hospital. You might encounter people you know from your town or area, both as workers and as patients. Of course, the local community hospital is your first stop if time is of the essence, whether you arrive under your own steam or by ambulance. If you turn out to have a more complicated situation or need a certain type of procedure, your doctors will *refer* you to a higher-level hospital. This referral happens all the time, if the equipment, technology, or staff at the community hospital cannot fix the problem.

Secondary Care Hospital

We hear less talk about the *secondary care hospital*, but it exists as an intermediate step between community and tertiary care. There is more specialized care than in the community hospital but not nearly what you will find in a tertiary care center.

Tertiary Care Hospital

A *tertiary care hospital* offers a variety of highly specialized services and equipment, in addition to general medical, surgical, and obstetrical care, and usually has many medical specialties represented. If your medical problem or type of surgery is complicated or high-risk, your doctors may refer or transfer you to this type of facility. Some examples of the kinds of services you might find in a tertiary care hospital are open heart surgery, organ transplants, a *neonatal intensive care unit*, and a level-one trauma unit. Some tertiary care hospitals also have *burn units.* There will be differences in the services offered between hospitals because certain tertiary care centers specialize in certain services while others specialize in different services. You will not find organ transplant services or burn units available at all tertiary care centers since these specialties require very specific resources and certifications, but you will likely find a neonatal intensive care unit (for high-risk pregnancies with possible complications for the mother or fetus) at all centers.

University Hospital or Academic Medical Center

A *university hospital* is integrally associated with a medical school. The physicians who practice here are also professors at the school. There is likely to be research activity as well at this type of hospital. A university hospital is always a teaching hospital because its mission includes training new physicians and other health care professionals.

Teaching Hospital

Many types of hospitals have a teaching component, from community up through highly complex university hospitals. Physicians, nurses, NPs, PAs and other health care professionals and personnel spend some time learning their craft in a classroom, but the real learning happens in the practice environment with actual patients. In a teaching hospital, physician trainees, called *residents* or *house staff or house officers,* will be involved in your care. In a *teaching hospital* you will also encounter medical students, nurse trainees, and other health professionals getting their hands-on real-life training.

Rehabilitation Facility (Rehab)

While the hospital is called an *acute care facility,* the *rehabilitation* center is associated with care for patients who need ongoing therapies but who do not require hospitalization. Rehab centers are *subacute facilities* that employ a host of health professionals under the direction of a physician. You will find occupational therapists, speech pathologists, social workers, psychologists, physical therapists, and physiatrists (rehabilitation doctors) at these facilities. The purpose of rehab is to restore patients to as high a level of functioning as possible before sending them home. Very often, patients who have such routine surgeries as hip or knee replacement will need a stay in rehab to learn new ways to use their muscles with a new *prosthetic* (artificial) joint in place. People who have had a stroke also often need rehabilitation, particularly if there has been significant damage from the stroke.

Skilled Nursing Facility (SNF or Nursing Home)

A *skilled nursing facility* is another type of subacute facility and is often housed in the same building as a rehab center. Many patients, particularly older ones, experience a steep decline in their general health as a result of being ill and being hospitalized. These patients might require a higher level of care than can be found at home or in the rehab center, such as IV medications, special feeding procedures, or close monitoring. Patients may be discharged to a skilled nursing facility even if they have been living at home prior to the hospitalization. Sometimes a stay in the SNF is temporary and is a transition to a major life change, requiring extra help and nursing visits at home. Other times, it is a semipermanent housing situation since, as a result of illness or age, patients cannot take adequate care of themselves. Patients with advanced dementia often require skilled nursing care.

LINKING YOUR INFORMATION: THE ELECTRONIC MEDICAL RECORD

Health systems and hospitals are undergoing another huge change in converting from paper charts or medical records into electronic media. As more and more hospitals adopt what is known as the *electronic medical record (EMR)*, there should be less need to repeatedly give your information about medical history and medications to various hospital staff along the chain. Your data or information will be entered into a computer, and then doctors and nurses and other health professionals who have authorized access can check your records to find out your status without having to ask you again. When the system works, there will be communication between different entities in a health system. So, for example, if you have multiple hospitalizations within one health or hospital system, your health care providers will have access to your previous health issues if you are readmitted. This system should make things easier, but as in all things technological, there are bound to be glitches and system outages. Further, many hospitals have not yet adopted this method of acquiring and sharing information. Since the manner in which your medical information gets passed along between medical professionals is critically important, we will have more to say about this in the chapters ahead.

CHAPTER 3

The Emergency Department Experience

WHY AM I NOT BEING SEEN? I WAS HERE FIRST

No place in the hospital is as baffling and as stressful as the emergency room (ER, but also called the emergency department, or ED). There are 136.3 million ER visits each year in the United States. Many patients without access to health care use the ER as their source of primary care. What this means is that people with many different kinds of health problems come to the emergency room: from children with stomach viruses to very sick or injured patients brought in by ambulance with major trauma, heart attacks, or strokes. Then there are the patients who have been sent in by their doctor to be admitted to the hospital through the portal of the ER. What a system! Understanding this system will be helpful in figuring out why, if you have arrived at 4:00 p.m., sent by your doctor who is concerned that you need to be admitted, you are still sitting in the waiting room at 10:00 p.m. and no doctor or nurse has seen you.

REGISTRATION AND TRIAGE

Registration and *triage* processes are different in every hospital, and the order in which events happen may vary. When you arrive at the emergency room, unless there is an extreme emergency, the first thing that happens is registration. In the registration process, information about name, address, next of kin, and insurance is collected. Once this process is complete, you may believe you are on your way to being seen by the medical staff. But in fact, early in the visit, a *triage nurse* will evaluate you to determine how serious the medical situation is and how quickly you must be seen by a physician or other health care provider. A level of urgency will be assigned. However, no matter what order is assigned to incoming patients, the minute a more seriously ill patient enters the emergency room door, the order can shift. Emergency room triage is not done on a first-come, first-served basis. Certain conditions warrant immediate medical attention. Severe trauma, heart attack, acute stroke, respiratory failure (difficulty breathing), and lack of consciousness are just some of the more serious conditions that will be tended to first. A long wait can be frustrating to a patient who is hurt or feels miserably sick. However, triage nurses are very good at their jobs and are specifically trained to make these decisions. They also have tools to evaluate the seriousness of the condition.

The only instance in which it might be advisable for you to be very assertive with the ER staff is if you or your loved one has experienced a major change in status since being triaged by the nurse while in the waiting room. Some examples might be loss of consciousness, trouble breathing,

TIP Speaking Up When Your Condition Has Changed or Worsened

If you or your family member suspects that there is a change in your condition that warrants immediate medical attention, it is appropriate to be proactive and notify the nearest medical professional or the clerk at the nursing station. This is the time to request that the nurse or medical provider return to the patient to determine if immediate intervention is necessary. You might say, for example, "I am here with patient X and we are very concerned that his condition is worsening." Here it is appropriate to be specific. If there is more bleeding or increased shortness of breath, say so. If there is a sudden dangerous situation (loss of consciousness, inability to breathe), please call for help in no uncertain terms. Remember that in your role as advocate for yourself or for your loved one, if there is legitimate concern, it is imperative that you be given the attention you deserve, and in the middle of a busy emergency department, you may have to ask repeatedly.

new chest pain, or major bleeding. At this point, someone—either you or your family member—**must** let staff know that there has been a change in your condition.

THE WORKUP

The *workup* is medical terminology for finding out what is troubling the patient. It is done through a variety of methods, which, taken together, give clues to the doctors, nurses, and other health professionals about how to *manage* (take care of) the patient. There are several elements to the workup: the all-important *vital signs* (from the Latin *vita*, meaning life), history taking, blood and urine samples, review of current medications, and imaging studies such as *X-ray*, *CT scan*, and *ultrasound* to obtain images of the patient's internal organs, muscles, bones, and tissue.

> **TIP**   Hand Washing
>
> Do not be afraid to ask if the person taking care of you, touching you or your medical equipment, has cleaned his or her hands. You might say something like, "I've noticed all sorts of signs suggesting I ask people if they have washed or cleaned their hands. I'm sure you have, and I didn't notice, but I would just like to make sure."

HISTORY TAKING IN THE ER—WHAT IS A HISTORY ANYWAY?

Along with information about current medications (see next topic), finding out about what health conditions you have is often the key to solving what landed you in the ER in the first place. Sometimes patients come in with obvious troubles. For example, if a person has been in a *motor vehicle accident* (MVA) and has cuts, bruises, or broken bones, the problems are evident to the staff and they will know what to do. However, for patients who have symptoms that can be caused by many different kinds of *underlying conditions* (existing medical illnesses), knowing about your history of illnesses, chronic diseases, or previous surgeries will help guide the medical professional in making decisions about what needs to happen next. For example, patients who have a history of high blood pressure are at greater risk for stroke or heart attack than other people.

Every clue that the doctors and nurses can gather is important. Essential information comes not only from how the patient is feeling at the moment and what the current *chief complaint* (the medical problem that causes an individual to seek treatment) is but also from the accumulation of illnesses or conditions in the past. Sometimes, particularly if you're feeling crummy, it's very annoying to have to tell about a surgery to remove your tonsils that happened fifty years ago. However, every question that is asked is intended to prompt you to reveal as much about your situation as possible.

Some patients with very complicated medical histories carry around typed pages that list their illnesses, date of diagnosis, and the names and phone numbers of the doctors who treat them for these conditions. Surgeries can also go on this list, along with the dates when they were performed. Many diseases or conditions seem to disappear for years but can recur, which is why knowing the date of occurrence matters so much. **The importance of a good history cannot be overstated.** The doctors and nurses really do want to hear details and in fact need to have them so that they can move ahead with the best possible care for you.

TIP   Before You Need to Go to the ER . . .

Put together a clear and concise medical history with dates, type of illness and surgery, and the names of all your doctors, including your specialist providers. Keep this list in your wallet for emergencies. Keep a separate list with your CURRENT medications—with doses. These simple preparations will save much time and aggravation during a stressful emergency room encounter.

MEDICATIONS AND MEDICATION RECONCILIATION

There is no way to exaggerate the importance of providing an accurate list of your current medications, herbal supplements, and even vitamin supplements. The best way you can help yourself or your family member is by maintaining a typed list of all current medications, the doses, how often you take them, and for how long you have been taking them. **This list should be kept in your wallet at all times.** If you do not have a list, try to remember to grab the medication containers or pill minders before you leave home, or the name and phone number of your pharmacy. These medications provide a tremendous amount of information to the physicians and nurses taking care of you in the hospital, particularly if they are meeting you for the first time. From your medication list, your hospital caregivers will be able to determine a great deal about your health conditions, including any chronic diseases you have.

Moreover, there are certain medications that will affect treatment decisions. Consider these common scenarios, which underscore why it is vitally important to maintain accurate and up-to- date lists of medications and doses.

Blood Thinners/Anticoagulants

Warfarin (Coumadin) is a *blood thinner* (also called an *anticoagulant*). This type of drug has been a lifesaver for people with *atrial fibrillation* (an irregular rhythm of the heart), stroke, blood clots, and certain kinds of mechanical heart valves. However, since it thins the blood, it has the tendency to make people bleed more than they would if they were not taking it. Therefore, medical staff must know if a patient is on blood thinners, especially in the case of trauma or if the patient must go to surgery. You also may require a different kind of medication or blood product to "unthin" your blood if you come in with a bleeding illness. Be sure you know why you are taking a blood thinner. What condition do you have that the blood thinner is treating?

The decision by a physician to *hold* (discontinue, at least temporarily) a blood thinner will vary according to the *indication* (reason) for which the thinner is given. It is considered much safer to stop a blood thinner if it was given for atrial fibrillation than if the patient has a mechanical valve in the heart.

Diabetes Medications and Insulin

Millions of people have insulin-dependent diabetes; if they were to come off their medications, serious health consequences would result. It is especially important for the doctor to know the kind of insulin, the dosages, and the last time it was taken. Many people who have diabetes take pills to help control their blood sugar. It is also critically important for the doctors and nurses to know about these medications, since some cannot be given during acute illnesses such as infection and heart failure. These medications may cause very low blood sugar if the kidneys are not functioning properly, and some may need to be held (discontinued or stopped) if a CT scan with contrast dye is required.

Antibiotics

The discovery of antibiotics has saved millions of lives by preventing life-threatening bacterial infections. Yet, as is the case with many medications, antibiotics may produce side effects. Most commonly, they are known to cause diarrhea but can sometimes have more serious side effects such as breathing problems. If a patient comes in with difficulty breathing due to an allergic reaction from an antibiotic, furnishing the information about the medication will save a great deal of diagnostic testing and unnecessary workup. Diarrhea, particularly that caused by the bacterium *Clostridium difficile* (commonly known as *C. diff*), can be a serious complication of antibiotic use in elderly people or in people with *compromised* (unable to fight off infections) immune systems (such as people with HIV and those having *chemotherapy*).

Blood Pressure Medications

Many blood pressure medications can affect both blood pressure and heart rate and therefore can result in multiple side effects such as fatigue and dizziness. The health care team needs to know about these medications and whether there have been any recent adjustments in the dosages.

Heart Medications

Some people have a condition called *congestive heart failure,* and many of them are taking multiple medications. Of particular concern to the health care provider is the "water pill"—often furosemide (brand name Lasix). This medication is often adjusted in the setting of *acute* (severe or sudden) shortness of breath and heart failure. It is critically important for the doctors and nurses to know what the patient's usual dose is.

Psychiatric Medications

People who have a history of common psychiatric illnesses such as depression and anxiety may be reluctant to talk to the health care provider about these medical problems because they feel embarrassed. Medical professionals are trained to understand that a psychiatric illness is a medical illness like any other. Because psychiatric illness is often treated with medications, and because these medications can lead to very serious side effects, including seizures, if stopped abruptly, medical professionals need to know about any psychiatric medications the patient is taking, and any recent changes in those medications or the doses.

Medication Reconciliation

Medication reconciliation as defined by the Joint Commission (a United States-based not- for-profit organization that gives accreditation to health care organizations) is "the process of comparing a patient's medication orders to all of the medications that the patient has been taking." This reconciliation is done to avoid medication errors such as omissions, duplications, dosing errors, or drug interactions. It should be done at every transition (change) of care in which new medications are ordered or existing orders are rewritten.

How Your Health Providers Ensure That You Are Taking the Right Medications

The process called *medication reconciliation* (called *medrec* in the hospital) means that all the patient's medicines, both prescription and over-the-counter (including supplements, vitamins, and complementary and alternative products), are listed in one place with dosing amounts and times so that the health care provider (and pharmacist) can look for possible interactions or mistakes in dosing and can avoid duplications of similar medication types. Patients frequently come into the hospital already on a regimen of drugs; some of these medications will remain, while others will be changed or eliminated, depending on the diagnosis. In addition, during the course of the hospital stay, you can expect to have your medications adjusted as new conditions are discovered and as you begin to recover. Medication reconciliation is an ongoing process that is refined continuously throughout the hospital stay.

This system of checks and balances is very important to protect your safety. Careful vigilance on your part and in collaboration with the doctors and nurses can often prevent overprescription of medicine, particularly after discharge. We urge you to become involved and to be aware of the list of your medications at every point along the continuum of the hospital stay and afterward. Do not forget to include any herbal supplements and vitamins that you are taking.

DIAGNOSTIC TESTS IN THE ER

Once the hospital staff has gathered information about the history and medications, it is likely that some kind of testing will have to be performed. Some of these tests are very benign, while others can be uncomfortable or *invasive*. Increasingly, patients are diagnosed in the ER through testing and imaging techniques. A doctor or other health care provider may or may not perform a physical examination right away; they may take a history and order diagnostic tests before examining you.

Below is a brief description of some common tests you might encounter in the ER, organized in alphabetical order after the all-telling and highly important vital signs. For a complete description of these and many more tests and procedures, please refer to chapter 8.

Vital Signs: Temperature, Blood Pressure, Heart Rate and Pulse Oximetry

Most likely, soon after you arrive, the triage nurse will perform this group of simple tests. Your temperature will be taken by mouth to see if there is a fever, a blood pressure cuff will be wrapped around your arm, and the nurse will listen with a stethoscope to hear blood pressure. Your wrist pulse may also be taken. *Pulse oximetry* will be performed on the finger to see if your blood has enough oxygen.

Other Tests

Blood Tests (Blood Work)
Often, **blood tests** will be done since there is a lot of information about the general state of health provided by the blood: signs of an infection, cardiac (heart) enzyme levels, anemia, liver problems, and elevated sugar are just a few of the conditions that can be diagnosed by the blood. Depending on what you have come in for, the blood tests might be very specific. Some blood results can be seen immediately, while others take hours, even days to be determined. In serious situations, treatment is never delayed while waiting for blood test results.

Radiograph (X-ray)
Radiographs (X-rays) are photographic images using electromagnetic waves to look at the internal composition of something. Any patient suspected of having a broken bone will undergo X-ray evaluation. Also, if you have severe abdominal pain, you may undergo an X-ray to look for a blockage in your gastrointestinal tract. It is standard policy in many hospitals for all adult patients getting admitted to the hospital to undergo a **baseline** (the first version of a test, against which future and subsequent versions will be compared) chest X-ray as well. The staff person who will administer the X-ray is called a **radiology technician** (or **tech** for short). You might be able to remain in your ER room or cubicle for this test if portable X-ray machines are available. If not, you will be transported to an X-ray room, where you will be given a heavy shield made of lead to protect the parts of your body that do not require imaging. You may be asked to lie down, sit, or stand, depending on the type of X-ray needed.

Computed Tomography (CT) or Computed Axial Tomography (CAT) Scan
A **CT scan** is useful as a way to see beyond what an X-ray can see. While an X-ray can usually determine if there is a broken bone, a CT scan can see inside to the internal organs. If you came to the hospital with trouble breathing, a CT scan of the lungs may be better able to see pneumonia, fluid in the lungs, or perhaps a **pulmonary embolism** (blood clot in the lungs) than an X-ray would. If you came to the hospital with abdominal pain, a CT scan may be better able to see a blockage in the intestines or inflammation or infection such as **colitis** (infection of the large bowel).

Depending on the reason or indication for your CT scan, the doctor may ask you to drink a large quantity of a flavored liquid. This substance is a contrast material that helps to differentiate the organs being viewed. The type of CT scan will be determined on the basis of the symptoms, suspected illness, and the safety of the test for you. If there is a problem with the kidneys, a CT scan with intravenous (IV) contrast might not be a suitable test. The doctor will make this decision after weighing all the pros and cons. Since CTs are made of many X-rays, there has been concern about exposure to too much radiation, which may be harmful. There have been tremendous improvements in reducing the amount of radiation for certain CT equipment; however, not all hospitals have acquired these newer machines. If you have had repeated CTs in the past, you may want to discuss with the doctor whether another technology form can be substituted.

Magnetic Resonance Imaging (MRI)

While CT scans are more suited for bone injuries, lung and chest imaging, and cancer detection, a *magnetic resonance imaging* test (*MRI*) is better suited for muscle, tendon, or ligament problems, spinal cord issues, and brain tumors. Fortunately, an MRI does not have the radiation exposure of a CT scan. Unfortunately, it usually takes about thirty minutes to perform, whereas a CT scan takes five minutes. In addition, many hospitals do not have open MRI equipment, and some patients find the closed MRI setup claustrophobic, since you are placed on a narrow board and your body is put through an imaging machine in a confined space.

Telemetry

Telemetry monitoring is continuous heart monitoring. The nurse will place stickers on your chest and limbs and will attach them to some kind of recording device. If your complaint is chest pain, it is likely that there will be telemetry monitoring. Other reasons for this monitoring include *acute heart failure exacerbation* (worsening of the heart's condition), *syncope* (fainting or passing out), or an *unstable arrhythmia* (abnormal heart rhythm).

Lumbar Puncture (Spinal Tap)

Lumbar puncture is a procedure in which a needle is inserted into the spinal canal to extract some fluid for analysis. It is useful to diagnose certain conditions such as meningitis and other infections of the central nervous system or brain. It has a reputation (which it has lived up to) for causing some discomfort, possibly pain, and it sometimes results in a headache after the procedure. A lumbar puncture can be performed by ER attending doctors, internists, and neurologists.

ER STAFF, CONSULTANTS, TECHNICIANS, AND SPECIALISTS

During your time in the ER, it may seem that an awful lot of people are coming to see you, ask you questions, and examine you. It may well be annoying and overwhelming and will add to the stress and discomfort you are probably feeling. The doctors, nurses, and other providers you meet in the ER are specially trained to take care of you. They are the first line of defense in the hospital and consequently are trained to see a wide spectrum of conditions and to think fast. In certain situations, in fact, they have to think very fast, since many patients come in with life-threatening conditions that require swift action. The triage nurses and registration clerks will see you first. It is unlikely that you will see them again once you have been put on the list to be examined.

Technicians and nurses will be in and out of your room or cubicle to draw blood, take X- rays, and check monitoring devices. Transport teams will wheel you to and from tests. Nurses will come in to check your vitals. If you are in a teaching hospital, medical students, residents, and fellows will precede the doctor (called an *attending*) to take a history and get the first look.

Although ER physicians are trained about a wide variety of conditions, there are several scenarios in which you can expect to see other types of doctors. Generally, what this means is that a *consult* will be called, and the other doctor will have to be located. Most of these other kinds of doctors are not part of the ER staff. Depending on the day and time, the consulting doctor could be in the hospital or possibly at some other location (outpatient office, operating room, or home). Some of these evaluations can be conducted on the phone or via video feeds.

In some hospitals the ER doctor does not have the authority to admit you but must confer with physicians in the department (or unit) to which you need to be admitted. For medical illnesses, these will be any of the medical specialties, including general internal medicine. For injuries and trauma or for emergency surgeries, it would be the surgery department, including the surgical specialties. What may be confusing is that within each department there are subcategories called divisions. Departmental and divisional organization varies greatly between institutions. For example, if you have a heart problem, you will be admitted to cardiology, which is usually (but not always) part of the medicine department. If you have a broken hip, you will be admitted to orthopaedic surgery, which is often (but not always) a division of surgery. In addition, related but separate specialties may be consulted. For example, if you've had a stroke, you will usually go to neurology, but a neurosurgeon's opinion may also be solicited. If you are a cancer patient, your own oncologist may want you admitted, but an internal medicine physician may already be involved. If this sounds confusing, that's because it is. In general, the larger the hospital, the more complex and more medical and surgical specialties there are.

Coordination and communication between the specialties is challenging in the ER and at other points during your stay. We discuss these issues in subsequent chapters and give pointers on how you, the patient, can facilitate communication among the health care professionals caring for you.

TIP Asking Staff to Identify Themselves

Do not be shy about asking the people asking you questions or taking care of you to identify themselves and their specific duty within the hospital. Generally, hospital staff will wear identification badges and they **should** introduce themselves. However, in today's busy medical world, this does not always happen. You have the absolute right to know who the person is in your cubicle or room. You can say, "It's nice to meet you. I am wondering how you are involved in my care." No one should be threatened by such an interaction, and you will go a long way in defusing what could be an awkward situation. In fact, you will be helping the staff person, and that alone will serve you well. Be sure to find out both first and last names.

TREAT FIRST, ASK QUESTIONS LATER

Emergency room doctors and nurses are trained to think and act quickly. If a serious condition is suspected, there will be no delay in treatment. It is possible that the treatment may be discontinued at a later point if it turns out that you're not affected by that specific problem. When it is determined that you do not have a specific problem, that is called *ruling out*. For example, a patient suspected of having meningitis is treated with antibiotics before the results of the *lumbar puncture* (spinal tap) are received, and any patient suspected of a serious *pulmonary embolism* (blood clot in the lung) is often treated with a blood thinner before the *radiographic studies* (series of images) are completed.

GETTING ADMITTED OR GOING HOME

A high proportion of patients (approximately 85 percent) will be sent home directly from the emergency room. These patients have been deemed not sick or injured enough to be admitted to the hospital. Many factors influence this decision in addition to the illness or condition that brought you in. A few of these factors include your age, your general state of health, and whether you have support from family or friends at home. Some hospitals have an intermediate step between admission and sending home. This would apply when you need to be watched (or monitored), stabilized, or treated briefly (see below for short-stay units) before being able to go home. If you have been to your doctor's office and he or she has sent you to the hospital for admission by calling ahead to alert the ER, then generally speaking, that clinical decision will be respected by hospital staff. However, given the recent changes in medicine, many primary care physicians no longer come to the hospital, and the decision regarding your stay can be made between the ER attending and a staff attending such as a hospitalist or surgeon.

As noted above, people with many different kinds of situations come into the emergency room. Sometimes, a *suture* (stitch) or two are all that is needed before you are sent on your way. Many people who appear very ill can be prescribed medication and sent home directly. About 15 percent of the time, the ER doctors in consultation with the family doctor, surgeon, or specialists come to the conclusion that you need to be admitted.

PAPERWORK AND MORE PAPERWORK

During the registration process, if your situation is not life-threatening, you will be asked to fill out forms or respond to questions about your personal information, and you will be expected to produce proof of insurance. If you do not have insurance, you may be asked to take responsibility for payment of hospital bills and associated costs of a stay. However, the 1986 Emergency Medical Treatment and Active Labor Act (EMTALA) law requires hospitals to treat and stabilize patients with emergency medical conditions regardless of ability to pay. If a decision is made for your admission, there will be more paperwork and forms, including *advance directives* (what your wishes are about being resuscitated) and health care proxy designees. Some states have forms for conditions of admission. This entire process of paperwork and providing information will vary from hospital to hospital and state to state.

SHORT-STAY UNITS (SSU)

Some hospitals have areas called *short-stay units*. In an effort to improve the flow through the ER and open up ER beds for new patients, these units are designed to provide less than twenty-four hours of care for those patients who are still having ongoing therapy or assessment but no longer need to be in the acute setting of the ER. Many patients after twenty-four hours in an SSU are discharged home. Others are officially admitted to the hospital for longer-term care. Most short stay units are designed and staffed with doctors and personnel to deal with specific diagnoses, such as chest pain, or specific populations, such as children or the elderly.

DELAYS IN GETTING A BED

The decision has finally been made to admit you to the hospital. Time to go up to your bed and get settled, right? Not so fast. Unfortunately, the reality is that it can take many hours from the time of admission to the time when you reach an assigned bed. There are many reasons for this. First and foremost, if a hospital is near its capacity, someone has to be sent home for a bed to open up for your admission. The discharge process for the patient who is leaving can take many hours. The attending doctor has to see the patient and write the discharge orders. The patient then has to either get a ride home or possibly be transported to a rehabilitation facility. Once the patient has vacated that bed, the room has to be cleaned and made sanitary again before you are placed there. Once a bed is vacant, there is also a rearrangement of already admitted patients to organize, or patients with similar conditions must be *cohorted* (grouped together). Many hospitals have daily "bed meetings" to oversee this process, with representatives from many different units in attendance. All this has to be done before you can get your bed, as it usually takes many hours to work up a patient in the ER.

Some other factors also include the time of day you are admitted and the time of year. During the late evening and the early morning hours, fewer staff members are available to get you through the testing and evaluation processes. A technician may need to be "borrowed" from another department. Doctors will need to be called in from the outside or pulled from looking after sick patients in other parts of the hospital. Not all of the testing machinery and equipment is operational during the night. Patients rarely get discharged overnight, so there are fewer vacated beds. The late fall and winter months (when the flu and other respiratory illnesses abound) usually have the longest wait times for a bed. Summer weekend evenings and holidays are notorious for an excess of trauma visits resulting from reckless behavior.

If you experience a delay in getting a bed after you have been admitted, do not feel discouraged or worried that you are not getting appropriate care. Hospitals are equipped to continue with a treatment plan no matter where you are currently resting.

Clinical Scenarios That Really Happen in the Emergency Room

ER Visit Take One

It is a sunny, late spring Saturday afternoon. An ambulance races up to the door of a large suburban emergency department. EMTs (emergency medical technicians) carefully but swiftly unload a stretcher with a middle-aged female dressed in jogging attire. She appears chalky in color and unresponsive. She is whisked through the ER doors and taken past triage, a waiting room filled with people, and put into a room near the nursing station for immediate evaluation. This patient has already started the process of being cared for in the ambulance because the situation appears dire. EMTs have likely called ahead to alert the coordinating nurse that a very sick patient is on the way. Emergency department attending doctors are at the ready to take charge. Gathering paperwork such as insurance information, history, etc., will take a back burner to immediate medical attention, as will other patients who arrived much earlier but with much less serious conditions. Soon the small critical care cubicle is filled with staff and equipment. There is organized chaos—the team is well practiced in resuscitating unconscious patients and stabilizing them for further evaluation.

ER Visit Take Two

Joe, a sixty-seven-year-old man with high blood pressure, comes into the emergency department because his stomach has been bothering him for a few days. In the last several hours, the pain has worsened and he has been unable to eat, drink, or concentrate on a TV program. Upon entering the ER he is first evaluated by the triage nurse, who asks him to state his problem and takes a quick set of vital signs. After it is determined that his abdominal pain is not critical in nature (unlike a heart attack, stroke, or a case of respiratory arrest), he is given paperwork to fill out and sent to the waiting room. After waiting for a couple of hours, he is taken into a room where he is first seen by a different nurse, who repeats his vital signs and takes a history. She then performs an EKG, draws blood to be sent to the in-hospital laboratory for analysis, and starts an IV (access for fluids and medication into the veins). Since this is a teaching hospital, an emergency room doctor in training (resident) is the first kind of physician to visit him. Joe will now finally get some pain medication. The resident takes another history and examines Joe. After the examination, the young doctor determines that Joe needs a CT scan to figure out the source of the pain. Joe is brought a container of oral contrast dye that he must drink before being taken to the CT scan room. He is transported to the scan room, where a technician administers the test, and is sent back to his cubicle. There is a long wait for the radiologist to read the results of the scan. He has now been in the ER for seven hours. At last, the results come back: he has diverticulitis (inflammation of spaces in the large intestine). Antibiotics will finally be started by IV, and a decision is made to admit Joe. The search begins for an empty bed.

CHAPTER 4

Getting Settled and Finding Your Way

YOUR HOSPITAL ROOM

Getting a bed in a room usually brings a sense of relief. You've got a place to put things down. There are chairs for family members to sit in. The bathroom is close by. You will have an option to pay for telephone and television hookups, good distractions for all. If you were admitted through the emergency department, you have left the chaos of the ER behind. If you have come from surgery, having been admitted earlier in the day, you will head to your room after a period in the *postanesthesia care unit (PACU, recovery room)*.

Now it is time to get oriented. When you get to your hospital room, the following things will happen:

You will meet your nurse and patient care associate (*nurse's aide*).
You will receive a demonstration of how your bed and all the switches and electronics work.
You may give a history and list of medications again if your hospital does not have your electronic medical record (EMR).
You will have your vital signs taken.
You will be weighed.
You may have additional lines and monitoring devices inserted or applied.
You will be asked to fill out a menu form to choose items for your next meal.
You will be given an opportunity to sign up for and pay for telephone and television service.

SAME-DAY ADMIT FOR SURGERY AND OTHER PROCEDURES

If you are scheduled for a surgery that is not urgent and if you have undergone *presurgical testing* (see chapter 13, about elective surgery), it is likely that you will not stay in the hospital prior to your operation. Instead, you will be asked to come to the hospital several hours before the scheduled time of surgery (this could be VERY early in the day since surgeons' first cases usually begin at 6:30 a.m.). Once you arrive, you will change into a gown, put on a paper hair cover, and remove jewelry, false teeth, eyeglasses, contact lenses, hearing aids, and any other prosthetic devices in preparation for administration of anesthesia and for surgery. After the surgery or other procedure is over, you will be *recovered* in the PACU. To be recovered means that you will be monitored very closely to ensure that you come out of sedation smoothly. The anesthesiologists and nurse anesthetists will usually accompany the patient to the PACU to help with the transition from the operating room or procedure room. The PACU has many nurses whose particular job is to watch patients after surgery and procedures. You will not be allowed out of bed on your own, and you will be hooked up to *drains,* IVs, and *monitors.* You will likely be quite groggy, possibly a little nauseated, depending on the kind of procedure and medications. Your family and friends will be able to visit you briefly in the PACU. You may not feel very friendly to visitors, but your loved ones will want to lay eyes on you and hold your hand.

When it is determined that you are sufficiently well or recovered enough to move on, you will be transported to your room. If you have undergone surgery or other major procedures, you will be confined to bed for several hours and will probably be groggy and lethargic. You may not be interested in television, and you won't be permitted to eat solid foods at first (see chapter 9, about nutrition in the hospital). Soon after surgery, you will be dependent upon nurses, aides, and family or friends to perform the simple tasks you take for granted when you are feeling well. Usually during the first twenty-four hours, after the nurses' status reports indicate readiness and the surgeon or physician deems it appropriate, you will be allowed—in fact, encouraged—to get out of bed and begin moving around.

UNPLANNED ADMISSIONS AFTER PROCEDURES OR OUTPATIENT SURGERY

Increasingly, minor surgeries are performed outside the hospital in *ambulatory surgery centers (ASC),* also known as outpatient surgery centers or same-day surgery centers. In addition, there are a variety of tests performed inside the hospital (examples: *endoscopy, colonoscopy, bronchoscopy, cardiac catheterization*) that use specialized equipment or require sterile conditions but do not require inpatient care. Occasionally, minor surgeries or other procedures and tests have unexpected results and complications, so instead of going home, you will have to be admitted to the hospital for observation, treatment, more tests, or further surgery. This is done at the discretion of the treating physician or surgeon and can be alarming for patients and family if you are unprepared. This happens about 5 percent of the time and occurs usually in older patients and mostly among patients receiving general anesthesia. The reason for hospital admission might also be as simple as the fact that the surgery occurred in late afternoon and the ambulatory surgery center closed up before you had adequate time to recover. Depending on where the patient is coming from and the arrangements with the hospital, admission can be directly to a room or through the portal of the emergency department.

YOUR ROOMMATES

Single Room or Sharing a Room

Depending on the space available and the possible need for isolation (see chapter 10, about protocols and precautions), you may be put into a single room. Otherwise, it's likely that you will share your room with another patient. You will be segregated by gender to avoid privacy issues and potential problems with bathroom sharing. (The option to pay extra for a single or private room does usually exist, so consider the private room if that is a high priority for you. Insurance companies will pay only up to a certain amount for hospital stays, and unless there is justification, a single room requires the patient to make up the difference.) While you may not relish the fact that you need to share a room, in previous decades (and indeed even currently in many other parts of the world) patient beds were lined up in large rooms where you might find twenty to forty patients together. These days, rooms hold between two and four patients.

In general, the higher the complexity level of the hospital, the more likely that you will room with a patient with medical or surgical issues similar to your own. For instance, in a community hospital, a patient in traction for a complex broken-bone surgery might share a room with a patient with pneumonia. In larger hospitals, however, patients are grouped by the *service* (medicine, surgery, neurology, etc.) they have been admitted to, so you will find patients who have knee replacements with other orthopaedic surgery patients, and patients with cardiac issues who require electronic and nursing monitoring will be housed together. This is another way in which efficiency is optimized, for different conditions call for different kinds of trained staff, different medical equipment, facilities, and different focus and attention to patient needs.

Rooms versus Wards

It is only in the last twenty years that patients were put into private or semiprivate rooms in hospitals. If you were hospitalized or visited an inpatient before that time, you will recall seeing beds lined up in a large room, separated by curtains. Patient wards are considered more efficient than separated walled rooms since they allow easier visual and physical access by staff to oversee patients; physicians and nurses claim to prefer a ward setup. The downside is the extraordinary loss of privacy and accompanying dignity experienced by patients. In the modern era there is greater focus on patient comfort and nourishing the "whole" patient to enhance healing, and so the concept of efficiency in this case has been overtaken by a more patient-centered approach. This is in contrast to the many ways in which the health care field seeks to streamline and move toward higher efficiency levels in many arenas, such as hospitalist physicians and electronic medical records.

Roommate Etiquette

Please be respectful of your room-mates, roommates' families, and friends. Follow the Golden Rule: do unto others as you would have them do unto you. What this means in very concrete terms is, do not allow your guests to overstay their welcome, leave garbage, carry on loudly, and let children run amok. Although your visitors may bring you distraction and relief, other patients may find them annoying. For privacy, make sure the curtain is closed. For discretion, keep voices down. For hygiene, don't let your guests use the patient bathrooms since they are designated for patient use only. (There are bathrooms for visitors in the hallways.)

Other examples of considerate manners include keeping radio and television volumes set to low or on headphones to avoid disturbing others and silencing the ringers on cell phones during the nighttime hours.

Occasionally there is an unfortunate mismatch of patients in a room. This could be as minor as a hard-of-hearing patient needing to raise the TV volume beyond what is tolerable. Or it could be something major, such as sharing a room with a terminally ill patient who is waiting for transfer to hospice care. Both of these scenarios can be very disturbing. We urge tolerance, forbearance, and understanding. Most patients are not purposefully upsetting or intrusive.

The New Reality: Cell Phone Access in Hospital Rooms

It used to be that the hospital disconnected your phone access after 9:00 or 10:00 p.m. to allow you to rest. For several years, cell phones were not allowed to be turned on in the hospital for fear they would interfere with monitoring equipment. Welcome to the new era: Almost everyone from six-year-olds to octogenarians carries a cell phone, and in most hospital areas they are permitted. Often patients do not even bother to get a hookup for the hospital landlines. The result of all this new technology and access is that phones ring and patients talk on the phone at all hours of the day and night and sometimes without concern for other patients. We urge you, your family, and your friends to be mindful of other patients' need for tranquillity. Many patients truly do need peace and quiet to cope with their illnesses and to recover.

If you should happen to be assigned to a room in which another patient's family is loud, unruly, or not observant of the rules, it is entirely appropriate to say something. You may start with the nurse. She will determine how to handle the other patient's family. If necessary, she will consult with a *nurse manager*, who has expertise in handling these types of situations. In extreme cases, if the situation persists, you may change rooms.

TIP   What to Do If You Have a Problem with Your Roommate

If your roommate is disruptive or has visitors who are too loud or inappropriate or stay too long, you may politely tell them that you would be grateful if they would try to keep it down since you require quiet. It is possible that they are not aware that they are causing you discomfort. Remember—being ill or recovering from surgery can be a time of great distress, and people tend to focus on themselves without meaning to be rude. If this does not produce results, then you must ask the nurse to intervene to enforce visitor etiquette or to help quiet a restive patient. Usually this is sufficient. However, sometimes a patient or family is extremely insensitive or obstinate and the nurse manager will have to step in. Generally speaking, nurse managers, by virtue of their job descriptions and demanding positions, are adept at handling "people problems." You can expect resolution. Nonetheless, if you are still very dissatisfied, you may ask to be moved to a different room. Hospital staff members want happy patients and families; it makes their jobs easier, and therefore, if it is possible, they will try to accommodate you as best they can.

Remember—if you feel it is justified, you may elect to request a private room, for which you will likely have to pay extra since insurance rarely reimburses for private rooms. Only you and your family can decide how important or feasible it is to afford this luxury.

The Roommate Problem

Uncle Phil had gone into the hospital for a simple valve replacement. He had great confidence in his surgeon and was at a topnotch hospital. A few days after surgery, his nurse noticed that one side of his face was drooping. She alerted the stroke team immediately, and Uncle Phil was whisked away for evaluation by a neurologist and interventional radiologist. Fortunately, there was minimal damage and the prognosis was good. However, instead of going home, Uncle Phil would have to go to stroke rehabilitation for two weeks to work on regaining movement in the affected side. Although this was not in the plan, he was a good sport about this change. When he got to his room at the rehab facility, however, he noticed a sign on the door saying that the patient with whom he would share the room had C. *diff.* and that gloves and gowns were required for all who entered. This was very distressing. It was bad enough having a prolonged time to recover, but Phil had heard about C. *diff.* and the diarrhea and misery it caused. He did not want to stay in a room with another patient with this highly contagious condition. He and his family contacted the nursing manager to insist that he be moved to a different room.

NAVIGATING THE UNIT

The Nurses' Station

The nurses' station is the central hub of the hospital floor, and by day it feels like a buzzing beehive. This is an area of high activity where staff members gather and interact. The entire functioning of a hospital ward or unit and coordination of patient care are controlled from the nurses' station, which is actually a misnomer since there are so many other professionals and staff who perform portions of their duties there. Unit clerks or secretaries are stationed at phones, patient call boards, and fax machines. There may be a hydraulic tube through which specimens and medications can be transported throughout the hospital. If there are paper charts, they will likely be located at the nurses' station on racks, shelves, or rolling carts. There will be a bank of computers nearby where staff can access patient information. On a large floor there will be more than one nurses' station, one for each area or section. Usually there are small rooms clustered around the nurses' stations where you will see physicians working on computers or charts, a locked medication room to which only nurses and certain other staff have access, the nurse manager or director's office, and a case-management/discharge-planning office.

Often, arriving visitors will check in at the desk for help locating a patient room. Physicians will conference with other physician specialists and nurses. In teaching hospitals, teams of residents and medical students will meet to begin *rounds* (time for officially seeing patients).

If you are in need of a service or have a question or request, it is likely that you will approach the nurses' station for assistance. You might ask when you will see your own doctor or find out when transporters will arrive to take you to a test or procedure. Or you might ask something as mundane as how late the cafeteria will be open. Whatever your need, please remember that hospital staff is usually engaged in vital patient care, and unless your request is urgent, you may have to wait a bit to get answers.

The Pantry

If your stay is more than a day or two, it is likely that you will want to find the pantry on your hospital floor. There often is a small room on your floor where patients, staff, and families can get water and ice and use a refrigerator or microwave. If you do avail yourself of the hospital refrigerator, please mark your items with your name and the date very clearly to avoid mix-ups about what belongs to whom.

The Linen Room

In some hospitals, instead of asking nurse's aides for bedding, pads, towels, blankets, and sanitary items, you are encouraged to help yourself to these items from the linen room if it is not kept locked or from a linen cart stationed in the hallway. Although bedding is changed regularly, you may need a fresh replacement because you may leak fluids or blood, have toileting accidents, or simply spill food or drinks. In addition, you and your loved ones may need extra blankets and pillows to stay warm and comfortable. If you ask at the nurse's station, you will find out if it is permissible to enter the linen room.

The Visitors' Lounge

Many hospitals have areas for visitors to gather while they are waiting to take a turn to see their loved ones. Patients who have doctor's orders to be out of bed will, if they're feeling up to it, visit with their friends and family in these lounges. Often a change of scenery is therapeutic for the patient and nicer for the visitors, away from the confinement of the hospital room. In days gone by, the visitors' lounge might have been called a *solarium*, a room or large porch in which patients might have been exposed to sunlight in a controlled environment as part of their therapy when they were not allowed outside. In line with more contemporary thought on fresh air and exposure to the elements, patients are no longer forbidden to be outdoors. Therefore, if there is outdoor space on hospital grounds and your physician gives the OK, it is acceptable for you to walk or be wheeled outdoors with family and friends.

VISITORS

Visiting Hours and Limits

Visiting hours are posted for a reason. Please have your guests respect them. It is not fair to other patients needing rest to have to deal with the noise, germs, and disturbance. It is disruptive and rude for your guests to be loud or inappropriate while visiting you in the hospital.

Who Should Visit?

Many hospitalized patients derive great benefit from the attention and care of visiting friends and family members. In addition to the comfort visitors bring, they may be indispensable as advocates and helpers when staff is busy with other patients. The decision about which and how many visitors is a highly personal one. Remember that it is not your job to entertain visitors if you are feeling poorly. Encourage friends and family who understand your needs, and discourage those visitors who may not be in tune with you.

Of course you want beloved children and grandchildren to bring joy to sick family members stuck in the hospital, but this is a decision that has to be carefully weighed:

1. Will the visit to an impaired or sick relative be frightening to the child?

2. Will it be worthwhile to expose a young child to the kinds of germs found in the hospital?
3. Is it fair to your loved one in the hospital or to other patients to be exposed to the many germs that kids may carry?
4. Does the child have enough self-control to maintain decorum and appropriate behavior while visiting?

Please think through this decision carefully.

TIP   Asking Staff to Wash Their Hands

Hospitals are hotbeds of dangerous germs. The kinds of "bugs" that proliferate are more dangerous here than in the community (outside world). If you read or listen to the news, you will have heard the terms *MRSA* (a kind of staph bacterium that does not respond to many antibiotics), *C. diff.* (a cause of serious and life-threatening diarrhea), and many other bacteria and viruses that may grow and spread in a health care setting. Keeping equipment and rooms clean in the hospital is a major focus. Yet patients remain at high risk from neglected hand-washing routines. Very often, fortunately, you will observe staff and providers going over to the sink and clearly washing up prior to examining you. However, if this does not occur, it is entirely appropriate, and very important, that you REQUIRE all staff and providers to wash their hands prior to putting on gloves before touching you. You will say, "Please wash your hands if you have not already done so." There is no need to apologize or explain. This is your absolute right. And it may save your life!

HISTORY AND MEDICATION RECONCILIATION AGAIN

Even though you will have been asked for a patient history in the ER, and maybe even more than once, it is likely that your nurse will take another accounting of your medications and history. This is an evolving field; ultimately the electronic medical record will save time and aggravation by transferring data seamlessly between departments. If your hospital does not have an electronic medical record, then you will find yourself repeating this very important information. Please remember that the emergency department does its very specific job and then passes along the patient to the admitting department. The admitting process often involves starting from scratch.

Therapeutic interchange means that a medication is substituted for another equivalent or similar medication. This happens when you are admitted on a medication that is not readily available in the hospital—not supplied by the hospital *formulary* (pharmacy). A pharmacist, physician, or nurse practitioner will rewrite the prescription such that you get the same *therapeutic value* (treatment by the medicine) as that from the previous medication. The new drug might be a generic, a different brand, or a drug in a similar therapeutic class that is supplied. It is important to note that you will most likely not experience any untoward effects from this substitution. However, in rare cases, a nonactive ingredient (a dye or coating, for example) may disagree with you or cause you to have a reaction. As in all things, it is important to let the medical providers know if something does not feel right. You might say, "I am not feeling quite right and wondering if any of my new or equivalent medications could be causing this problem."

CHAPTER 5

Figuring Out the Care Team

A key step in getting settled is figuring out who the care team is. There are all kinds of staff persons in various uniforms. You will see people in white coats of all lengths (short white jackets often, but not always, signify medical students), scrubs in many colors, staff wearing street clothes, and combinations of all of the above. Making sense of all these hospital workers with different functions can be very challenging.

There was a time, not so long ago, when there were fewer health care professionals in the hospital; their uniforms communicated their function, and the hierarchy was very clear. Those days are gone, and they are not coming back; there are a myriad of professionals, paraprofessionals, other health care workers, and professions in the hospital. Much of the formality of a strict hierarchy is gone. Previously, nurses could be identified by their white uniforms, white hosiery, white oxfords (NOT sneakers!), and starched white caps. When is the last time you saw a nurse wearing a cap? Now nurses often wear colorful scrubs and smocks. You will see them wearing clogs or sneakers—after all, they are on their feet most of the day. Older individuals will also be surprised to note the presence of male nurses, since a career in nursing was traditionally a female-dominated profession. Although the field is still approximately 90 percent female, there is a growing trend for men to enter into nursing; it is a respected career choice.

Stethoscopes too connoted something very specific—doctors and only doctors draped stethoscopes around their necks. Now many kinds of health care professionals sport stethoscopes, and often the work previously done by stethoscope is done electronically by telemetry monitoring.

You Can't Tell a Book by Its Cover

Often when rounding in the hospital on the weekends as a hospitalist, I would dress differently than I did during the workweek. Putting in a twelve-hour day and often being responsible for supervising rapid responses for very ill patients, I would wear scrubs instead of my normal professional dress. Even though I always displayed my ID badge, I was often mistaken for a different member of the health care team, not the medical attending physician. Particularly as a female, I was often asked if I was the nurse, the physical therapist, nutritionist, or social worker— all traditional female fields. Do not assume you know the professional role of the individual entering your room on the basis of how they are dressed. Always be sure to ask who they are and to define their role in your care—*Karen Friedman*

White Coat Mystique

In previous years, a starched long white jacket on a serious individual meant DOCTOR!!! Nowadays, many health care professionals wear white coats: nurses, pharmacists, physician assistants, social workers, etc. This trend makes it difficult to sort out the type of professional with whom you are interacting. Some people find the white coat threatening, harking back to the day when doctors had an absolute authority that was never to be questioned. You may notice that often the professionals who take care of children do not wear white coats but choose whimsical smocks or street clothes to greet their little patients. Here are two key guiding principles: (1) nothing about your hospital stay should be intimidating, and therefore we urge you to ask questions about all of your care processes; and (2) white coat or not, every individual with whom you have ANY interaction should identify himself or herself to you.

THE NURSE IS KEY—WHICH ONE IS THE NURSE ANYWAY?

Nurses are highly trained professionals, who have spent a long time in school learning about the human body and how to take care of patients.

Nursing has become a very specialized field, and nurses work in different areas that all require specific skills—some of which your physician may not have. Your nurse has tremendous responsibility in terms of monitoring you as a patient, administering your medication, and maintaining accurate documentation that guides the treatment and planning of everyone who takes care of the patient. Today's nurses are a highly valued component of the care team; they are on the front lines of patient care and participate with other providers in making care decisions. The old model of subservience to doctors has disappeared. In its place is a new model of empowerment, professionalism, and interprofessional practice.

Identifying the Nurse/Nurse's Aide Team

Some hospitals will have a white board with the name of the nurse and nurse's aide filled in for that shift. This is a good place to start, as most interactions will occur with these individuals.

Shift Changes

What may be confusing is that you might see your nurse for one

Nursing Burnout

Nurses have tremendous responsibility in delivering patient care, documentation, administering medications, and monitoring a patient's evolving condition and response to treatments. They typically work long—often twelve-hour—shifts and as a result, may suffer from fatigue and stress. Patient care is demanding and constant, and the job, although rewarding, is arduous. Further, there are nursing shortages, which put tremendous pressure on existing nurse staffing. Years of this kind of work take a toll, and the result may be a kind of mental, physical, and emotional exhaustion, which is termed *nurse burnout*. The consequences of nurse burnout impact the nurses themselves, their families, and their patients. Various national organizations and nursing advocacy groups are working diligently to prevent burnout by increasing staffing ratios at the organizational level and providing support at the personal level.

twelve-hour shift and then not again during the entire hospital stay. If you are lucky, you will have the same nurse for a couple of days in a row.

More likely than not, you will have several different nurse/nurse's aide teams taking care of you during your stay.

Nursing Reports

Between shifts, your nurse will *give report* to whoever is taking over for him or her. This is termed a *patient handoff*, defined as one health care professional communicating all the information relative to the patients whom he or she cared for during the previous shift. During this report a nurse will relay what changes have occurred, go over your medications, your current status, and whatever protocols are in place or special concerns you might have. Depending on whether there are paper records or electronic records, documentation is the cornerstone of nurse-to-nurse communication (as it is between all health care professionals). Nursing report is a lengthy and comprehensive process; however, sometimes details can be left out. This is where your role as an advocate comes in handy. When the next shift nurse introduces herself or himself to you, you will have the opportunity to check that she or he has learned the particulars of your situation. This situation does not have to be specific to medical information. For example, if your loved one in the hospital is inclined to get out of bed on his or her own, and there is reason to believe that this is not safe (because of the risk of falling), then it is incumbent upon you to stress that your loved one needs assistance. This information may or may not have been recorded or previously communicated, and therein lies the problem. In the absence of knowing with certainty that a key fact has

Relationship-Based Care

Relationship-based care incorporates patient priorities into the traditional nursing-patient interaction by involving the patient and family in care processes. There are three principles of relationship-based care: (1) care of the patient; (2) care of self—the nurse's accountability for his or her practice; and (3) care of colleagues, fostering mutual trust and respect between nursing team members. This approach has been shown to support and empower nurses, as it encourages open dialogue. Patients report that the nurses were "talking with me, not about me," which helped them feel less anxious about their care.

been related to your care provider, it is always safer and better for you to succinctly relay important information.

There is tremendous variation—even within one hospital—about how nursing reports are given. Sometimes there will be a general preshift meeting at which there will be updates with the entire nursing staff to go over patient information. This will usually be led by a nurse manager, or *charge nurse*. At this level, only the broadest topics will be covered, without getting down to the nitty gritty. There might be a discussion of patients being discharged, patients going to hospice, or any special education programs occurring during the shift.

Increasingly, as there is a focus on what is termed *relationship-based care*, the traditional patient handoff will migrate to the bedside, where the patient and family may participate in the handoff process, providing key information and filling in the gaps.

TIP   Relationship-Based Care

If you are fortunate enough to encounter this innovative approach at your hospital, it would be another opportunity for you to take a proactive role in your care. Even if this practice is not adopted in your area, you might take a very proactive stance and request that the handoff occur at the bedside and with your participation.

Nurse's Aides/Patient-Care Associates (or Assistants)

Nurse's aides are called by different names in different hospitals, and you will likely be seeing many of them. They work in tandem with the nurse assigned to you and take care of routine matters, some of which were previously the domain of nurses. Nurse's aides, or *patient-care associates (PCAs)*, have some training but not nearly as much as nurses. Nor do they require licensure. You will encounter them when they come to draw blood and take vital signs (i.e., temperature, pulse, and blood pressure). They will also perform personal hygiene tasks such as bathing and helping with toileting. They change linens and bring fresh hospital gowns.

Nurse Managers

Your nurse, nurse's aide, and probably many other workers on the hospital unit, depending on how the hospital is organized, report to and are supervised by a nurse manager. She or he oversees all aspects of the care team, coordinates with the doctors, and maintains responsibility for the smooth operation of a hospital unit (floor or ward). In short, the nurse manager is the boss. If everything proceeds smoothly, you may never get to meet her or him. However, as we know, sometimes things do not go according to plan, and there are problems that cannot be solved without the help of the nurse manager. She or he will intervene if trouble is suspected. A good nurse manager has eyes and ears out in every room and will know when trouble is brewing. If you have a roommate with whom you absolutely cannot get along or you have a major complaint about your care, you should contact the nurse manager. Generally, the nurse manager is put in this job because she or he has the ability and the personality to smooth over situations and to ensure that staff is doing what they need to be doing.

TWO "NEW" PROVIDER TYPES

Physician Assistants

Physician assistants, or *PAs,* are another type of medical professional. They are trained to obtain medical histories, perform examinations and

TIP Communication between Health Care Providers

Always be proactive and assume that your doctors and nurses have not been put in touch with each other. This is important not only at discharge but also at shift changes. You might say, "Nurse, what did my doctor say when you spoke with her this morning?"

procedures, order treatments, diagnose illnesses, prescribe medication, order and interpret diagnostic tests, refer patients to specialists as required, and first-assist in surgery. Physician assistants, sometimes known as doctor's assistants, are individuals who practice medicine under the supervision of a physician.

TIP   PA and NP Credentials

If you are puzzled about the different designations and initials after the names of your providers, look for these credentials in the form of initials:

Here is how to identify a physician assistant: PA (physician assistant), PA-C (certified by the National Commission on Certification of Physician Assistants), RPA (registered physician assistant), RPA-C (registered and certified physician assistant), APA-C (physician assistant trained by the army as a flight surgeon), PA-S (student physician assistant in training).

Nurse practitioners may have their specialty designated as part of the initials. Here is how to identify a nurse practitioner: FNP (family health), ACNP (acute care), ANP (adult), PNP (pediatrics), PMHNP (psychiatry and mental health), NNP (neonatology), GNP (gerontology), WHNP (women's health).

Although PAs' training method is similar to that for physicians (classroom plus practical training after four years of college), the training is much shorter for PAs than for MDs. PAs sometimes are required to have a master's degree, depending on the state in which they practice. They are a somewhat new hospital professional. They are integrally involved in patient medical and surgical care in today's hospital world.

Nurse Practitioners

A *nurse practitioner,* or *NP,* as they are often called for short, is an advanced practice nurse (APN) who has completed graduate training in the form of a master's or doctoral degree. Nurse practitioners are registered nurses who have received extra education and training in areas that were traditionally reserved for physicians. Some NPs have worked as registered nurses for many years. Some have never worked as a registered nurse and have gone through an accelerated program that focuses on skills and knowledge traditionally reserved for physicians. They thus have different expertise, knowledge, and practice ability in certain medical areas than RNs do.

To become licensed to practice, nurse practitioners have to pass national board certification in an area of specialty (such as family health, women's health, pediatrics, adult health, acute care), and they are licensed through the state nursing boards rather than medical boards. Special focuses of the nurse practitioner field are individualized care, the effects of illness on the lives of the patients and their families, and patient education about wellness and prevention.

NPs can serve as a patient's primary health care provider. They can treat patients of any age if they have licensure to do so. In some states nurse practitioners can work independently of physicians, while in other states, a physician must supervise the NP's practice. Like PAs, NPs are integrally involved in patient medical and surgical care in today's hospital world.

TIP Asking Staff to Identify Themselves

Do not be shy about asking people who are taking care of you to identify themselves and their specific duty within the hospital. Generally, hospital staff will wear identification badges, and they **should** introduce themselves. However, in today's busy medical world, this does not always happen. You have the absolute right to know who the person is in your cubicle or room. You say, "It's nice to meet you. I am wondering how you are involved in my care." No one should be threatened by such a mannerly interaction, and you will go a long way in defusing what could be a tense situation. In fact, you will be helping the staff person, and that alone will serve you well. Make sure to get first and last names. It's useless to know that your nurse's name is Judy; you need to know her last name as well.

TYPES OF HOSPITAL PROFESSIONALS AND STAFF

Following, in alphabetical order, are other hospital professionals, paraprofessionals, and workers you will encounter.

Clergy, Chaplains

Pastoral support and consultation may be offered by the hospital itself or with allied organizations. Hospitals with religious affiliations will certainly have floating chaplains who will be available to help patients and families deal with illnesses and death. The usual garb associated with each religion will help identify the affiliation: priests wear collars, rabbis wear yarmulkes, Eastern Orthodox priests wear long black robes, and Muslim imams wear long robes and skullcaps and are usually bearded. The Protestant denominations will be more difficult to spot.

Interns in Many Professions

Whether bedside RNs or NPs, nurses increasingly have one-year residency programs. So do those getting PhDs in psychology and other fields. You may thus hear the term "resident" or "intern" applied to a trainee in nursing or psychology or another health profession. This educational method is a good thing but can make for a confusing situation in which it is difficult to sort out the roles and care responsibilities of so many individuals.

Dietary Worker

The dietary worker is the person who brings the tray of food up from the hospital cafeteria, usually on a large pushcart. In most hospitals you will be asked to fill out your preferences and choose menu items, according to your dietary needs and restrictions. If there is a problem with the type of food brought, you can start by asking this hospital worker to make changes.

Dietitian (and Nutritionist)

A registered *dietitian (RD)* is a professional who has had education and training about human physiology and nutrition science. *Nutritionists* may also be involved in this process; they have less formal training and regulation than dietitians (requirements vary from state to state). These individuals will consult with the other members of the health care team to determine the type of diet patients should have. We explore this topic very fully in chapter 9.

Discharge Planner (Case Manager)

You may never meet your *discharge planner*, also called *case manager*, but you should be aware that from the moment you are admitted, someone, usually a nurse, is figuring out your *discharge disposition* (where you go after the hospital). A discharge planner works with rehabilitation centers, nursing homes, hospice facilities, and even the transportation companies to ensure that you will be properly sent home or to the next stop in your recovery. Patients who are well enough will be discharged to home. We will discuss the discharge process and planning in great detail in chapter 15.

Environmental Worker (Janitor)

The work of keeping hospitals clean is critical in making sure you are in an environment that is not only pleasant but also safe. Bandages, tubing, and other medical detritus must be carefully and safely disposed of—and not just to protect patients and others who work in the hospital but to protect the broader community outside the hospital.

Cleaning hospitals is not like cleaning a home. It takes very specialized effort to not only keep hospitals clean but also prevent the spread of infection. The role of *environmental workers* is to use their knowledge and training to keep the patient and staff areas and offices and laboratories clean and disinfected. Under the supervision of nursing staff, environmental workers will sanitize a patient room after the patient has been discharged. This is a specific process that employs potent antibacterial and antiviral chemicals.

Orderly or Transporter

Orderlies transport patients from one area to another area; from rooms to tests, surgery, dialysis, and imaging; and then back to rooms, as appropriate. These are typically unskilled workers, but they still have to undergo extensive training to handle patients and must be educated to observe all safety and privacy protocols.

Pharmacist

In an era in which there is great focus on patient safety and avoiding medication errors, we have seen more and more *pharmacists* integrated into the day-to-day activities of patient care; these professionals are termed clinical pharmacists. You may see them making rounds by the bedside with the doctors and nurses. The training for clinical pharmacists is similar to that for the professional you encounter in your local drugstore but with a special focus on patient care. These days, pharmacists graduate from training with a Pharm D (doctor of pharmacy degree), so it is appropriate to address them as Dr. Clinical pharmacists have had postgraduate education and residencies in a general or specialty track field (such as oncology) and have gained knowledge in biomedical, pharmaceutical, and sociobehavioral sciences.

Phlebotomist

Phlebotomists have had training to draw patient blood. In some areas, this requires licensing. Most often, the phlebotomist collects blood by *venipuncture* (drawing blood through a vein), but for very small quantities, he or she will perform a finger stick, or in infants a heel stick. With special training, phlebotomists may collect blood samples from arteries (for *arterial blood gas* tests).

Physical Therapist (PT)

Physical therapists, also called *PTs*, are highly trained individuals concerned with helping patients move and regain mobility. They have had extensive education about human anatomy and structure and function of our moving parts, as well as practical internships, working with patients during a hospital stay. In certain parts of the hospital—where orthopaedic surgery or stroke patients are admitted, for example—they are key personnel who take a strong role in motivating patients to move around prior to discharge. Although much of their work with these patients occurs on the outside, after discharge, PTs are also very important in stroke recovery. You might see a PT helping a patient along a hallway, propping the patient up and giving encouragement. In fact, studies document that patients usually have faster recoveries if they are mobilized early in their hospital stay (see sidebar on bedrest in chapter 10). PTs employ their skills to make sure that patients get out of bed, and instruct aides and family members to help patients become mobile. Many patients will need to be seen by a physical therapist during their stay to determine the discharge disposition based on their physical abilities. The PT can assess whether a rehabilitation facility is needed.

Respiratory Therapist (RT)

Respiratory therapists help take care of patients with lung problems. You will see them with the following designations: certified respiratory therapist (CRT), registered respiratory therapist (RRT), or certified respiratory therapy technician (CRTT). They are trained professionals with degrees and credentialing to educate patients and manage airway issues. In the hospital setting, RTs work alongside their colleagues and are called upon to give medications and administer treatments for patients with cardiopulmonary disease. They are integrally involved with critical care medicine, where they may insert tubes, lines, and catheters (see chapter 11, about intensive care units). Respiratory therapists are also involved in assessing whether patients are taking in enough oxygen and in administering oxygen when it is needed. A respiratory therapist will also assist the anesthesiologist, in which case he or she will monitor and regulate breathing for the patient during surgery. If there is a respiratory care unit, RTs manage the day-to-day care of patients on *ventilators* (breathing machines). Usually RTs are organized as part of the pulmonary and critical care departments in a hospital. RTs generally make treatment decisions in consultation with physicians and surgeons.

Social Worker or Patient-Care Advocate

A *social worker* will step in when patients appear to need extra help adjusting to their illness, if there has been a significant change in the patient's status, if there is evidence that the patient's inability to care for himself or herself or the family's inability to take care of the patient played a part in the patient's hospitalization. A good example might be a patient with diabetes who is unable to self-inject with insulin. Another common scenario is an older patient living alone who forgets to take his medication. Hospital social workers are professionals, often with master's degrees, denoted as MSW. They will ensure that the patient has good *social supports* (network of family and friends) on the outside, and they will be instrumental in setting up those networks through local social services when there are gaps.

Unit Clerk

Do not underestimate the role and the importance of the *unit secretary,* or *unit clerk.* This individual functions as the "brain" of the floor or unit, and a good unit clerk keeps things humming with admirable efficiency. A unit clerk—particularly in high-traffic, high-volume areas of the hospital—coordinates the flow of patients, transporters, reports, charts, and all personnel across the unit. It is frequently a challenging juggling act, which requires patience, a high degree of organization, and good people skills, for the unit clerk, although technically reporting to the nurse manager, must answer to virtually every person who passes through his or her unit. The unit clerk will often be the first individual you encounter when you enter a hospital unit; he or she will sit front and center at the nursing station, which is the traditional activity hub.

Volunteer (Formerly Candy Striper)

Remember the days when eager young ladies in adorable pink outfits offered acts of kindness around the hospital to grateful patients? Well, you may still find them, especially in the summer, but more than likely you will see kindly pink-jacketed senior citizens and individuals of all ages seeking to add purpose and meaning to their lives by volunteering in the hospital. You may see volunteers pushing magazine racks, leading therapy animals, or simply greeting visitors who come into the hospital. They are a welcome and necessary addition, often fulfilling the duties that increasingly overworked staff cannot get to. Moreover, they contribute to the cheerful ambience in an otherwise somber setting. There are other types of volunteers as well. Aspiring medical students will often do a stint of volunteer work, helping physicians with research or chart work. These days becoming a hospital volunteer is not a casual process. Individuals wishing to donate their time must take courses about safety, decontamination hazards, fire safety, and patient privacy protocols. They must also have all their immunizations and tuberculosis testing up to date prior to beginning work.

GETTING THE ATTENTION OF BUSY HEALTH CARE PROFESSIONALS AND STAFF

It is important to remember that most of the health care professionals you will encounter in the hospital have chosen to embrace a lifetime of work in a caring profession. Health care professionals and others who work in health care are invested in decreasing suffering and curing medical problems. The modern landscape of health care is ever more demanding and stressful, with an explosion of information coming at both providers and consumers every day.

> **TIP** Getting the Attention of Your Health Care Providers and Professionals
>
> If your health care providers in the hospital appear harried and overwhelmed and you have difficulty in getting their attention, it is not because they do not want to provide topnotch care but because their workload is very large. Nonetheless, you have the right to have their full attention, and you must always make your needs very clear. You might say, "I would like to hear an updated report on how I am doing (or when a test will occur, or when discharge will happen). Can you please tell me what time I will see you later to find out this information?"

You may have noticed—since you are at the end of this chapter—that we haven't mentioned doctors. In the modern medical era with so many specialties and subspecialties, different training levels, and rapid hospital organizational change, the roles and descriptions of physicians are very complex. Therefore, we have decided to dedicate a separate chapter to that discussion. Please see chapter 6.

CHAPTER 6

Physicians of All Kinds

THE QUARTERBACK, OR WHO'S IN CHARGE?

Over and over patients tell us that they are frustrated because they have trouble identifying the medical expert in charge of the case. Furthermore, it seems as though specialist physicians sometimes do not communicate with each other about patients whose care they share: one hand does not know what the other is doing. Here is some background: the more complicated the case and patient's situation and the more extensive the *co-morbid conditions* (illnesses in addition to the ones for which a patient is admitted), the more physicians are involved. In large medical centers where there are *superspecialists*, you may find five or six doctors ministering to different organ systems and parts of your body. Clearly this is a different model from the old image of the friendly GP with the black bag who took care of your whole body. We acknowledge the problem of the number and array of health care providers and specialists and the confusion it gives rise to, and while we do not have a solution, we'd like to offer some suggestions:

1. Although it may appear that your doctors are not communicating with one another, they will be reading your chart, whether paper or electronic, to see their colleagues' comments and what procedures and medications have been ordered. However, in the spirit of taking nothing for granted, you might say when the

pulmonologist (lung doctor) stops by, "Dr., have you seen what my *cardiologist* has to say?"

2. If you happen to be in a hospital where there are *hospitalists*, there's your quarterback. He or she will coordinate with the different specialists and will function as the go-to physician, even if a specialist trumps the hospitalist in the pecking order.

3. If the doctor who admitted you actually *rounds* (officially sees patients) in the hospital (as opposed to dropping by as a friend or a comfort), then he or she will be in charge.

Residents and *fellows* (and *NPs* and *PAs*), no matter how confident they appear, how many orders they write, and how often they see you, are NEVER in charge of your case. Residents and fellows are doctors in training. Nurse practitioners and PAs are nonphysician providers and may be supervised by an attending physician. Attending physicians are always in charge of your case. You may find residents very accessible; they are a huge resource when you need to ask questions about your care, your tests, and your medications. NPs and PAs have put in years of training and may have spent long hours with you, and they are very knowledgeable about your care. Remember that health care professionals work as team, with your care and well-being at the center.

Sometimes, during the hospital stay, there will be a change in the physician and specialist taking care of the patient. This is because it is not always immediately known what kinds of services and doctoring a patient will need, even if it is evident that the patient needs to be in the hospital. Suppose, for example, that a patient comes in with chest pain and is admitted by a medical doctor such as an internist. After initial tests are run and are returned positive for a heart problem, a cardiologist will become involved in the care. Now suppose that the patient's symptoms and tests indicate that he or she needs to go to the ***cardiac catheterization lab*** (the unit where there is equipment that enables the doctor to see the blood vessels around the heart) to explore with ***angiography*** (a test involving dye that shows the veins, arteries, and heart chambers) whether the arteries are open or ***occluded*** (blocked). This is a job for an ***interventional cardiologist***. Let's now suppose this patient's coronaries are extremely occluded, and it is determined that surgery is needed. Enter the ***cardiothoracic*** surgeon. As you can see, the care of the patient has passed from one specialist to another as the need arose.

> **TIP**   Finding Out Who's in Charge
>
> It will be important to know the doctor who has the ultimate responsibility for your care. This is because this physician will likely coordinate with other consultants and will be the key decision maker for your management. If there are many specialists consulting on your case or if you have changed services or moved to a different level of care, this may be very confusing. If you are in a teaching hospital, the doctor in charge will not be the resident or the fellow. Be sure to ask your doctors and nurses the name of the doctor who is specifically in charge of your care and to keep you informed if there are changes during your stay.

So Many Kinds of Doctors Taking Care of Different Medical Problems

Aunt Gertie was getting ready for a big Sunday family dinner with all the family and grandnephews. She was very excited to see everyone and was planning to outdo even her previous cooking efforts. So much to do, to clean, to prepare, to set the table, and what to do first? She was rushing around to put the best china on the table when her foot caught the corner of the rug in the dining room. Before she knew it, she was just like the woman in the TV commercial—she had fallen and she couldn't get up. Luckily for her, her nephew Tommy was coming over early to help out. As soon as he saw her on the floor, he picked her up to bring her to the emergency room. Gertie was in pain, confused, and a little woozy. The doctors examined her and wanted to do some tests. After what seemed like a long wait, she arrived at her room. A hospitalist doctor from internal medicine (just like her GP) stopped by to tell her that her sugars were high and her blood was very thin from the warfarin she was taking for her heart problem. The next day, an orthopaedic surgeon stopped by to say that the X-rays showed a broken hip. Now HE was going to be her doctor and wanted to operate to fix the hip. This was very confusing for Gertie. Who were all these different doctors? She wanted one doctor to take care of her, not many. Tommy came to the rescue once again. He asked Gertie's nurse to give him the name and telephone number of the surgeon who would be in charge.

Attending Physician

The attending physician is the doctor in charge of your care. Traditionally this doctor would have been your primary care doctor, who knows you from the *community* (where you live, if it is not in a skilled nursing facility). As health care is changing, however, this is no longer the norm. More commonly now you will receive care from someone called a hospitalist. A hospitalist is a trained internist or family practitioner who mostly cares for hospitalized patients as the attending physician and generally has either a small or no outpatient practice. Hospitalists will care for you in the hospital and will be in communication with your primary care provider on the outside, if you have one. If you do not have a primary care provider, the hospitalist will help you to find one prior to discharge and pass along your information to that provider. Increasingly, and to maximize efficiency, there are other types of hospitalists who take care only of inpatients—for example, you might encounter neurology hospitalists or pediatric hospitalists.

Specialist

Specialists are doctors who spend extra time in training after residency (*fellowship*) to concentrate on a specific kind of medicine or surgery field.

The attending physician may require expert guidance from physicians in other fields depending on the patient's medical problems. This is a called a *consult*. For example, if you have a severe infection, the attending may ask for the help of an infectious disease doctor. The infectious disease doctor is the specialist who will make recommendations to the primary team—which includes the hospitalist. The primary team will review the recommendations of the specialist and discuss those recommendations with you to determine the best course of action. Some patients will not have any specialist care, and others will have many—depending on your condition and also the complexity of the hospital. Your attending physician is responsible for coordinating all the different recommendations to the primary team.

Here are some specialists you might see: a *cardiologist* if there are heart problems; a *pulmonologist* if there are lung issues; a *nephrologist* if there are problems with your kidneys; a *gastroenterologist* if there are problems with your stomach, liver, or intestines; a *neurologist* if you have had a stroke or a movement disorder such as Parkinson's disease. If you have a cancer diagnosis, either previously diagnosed or discovered during the inpatient stay, it will often require a consult by an *oncologist*. Sometimes these specialists will be doctors you know and who have cared for you on the outside as an outpatient. This will occur if the specialist has *privileges* at the hospital where you are admitted. Otherwise, the consulting specialist may be a doctor you have not met before.

There are different kinds of surgeons who may be called to consult, depending on what type of surgery is needed. In addition to general surgeons, here are some surgical specialists: *orthopaedic surgeons*

Providers

Primary Care Provider

An internist, either MD (medical doctor) or DO (doctor of osteopathy); family practitioner (FP); nurse practitioner (NP); or physician assistant (PA)

Specialist—in Any of the Subspecialties of Internal Medicine

Allergy and immunology, cardiovascular disease, critical care medicine, endocrinology, diabetes and metabolism, gastroenterology, geriatrics, hematology, hospice and palliative medicine, infectious disease, nephrology, oncology, pulmonary disease, rheumatology, and sleep medicine

Surgical Specialties (Recognized by the American College of Surgeons)

Cardiothoracic surgery, colon and rectal surgery, general surgery, gynecology and obstetrics, gynecologic for bones and cartilage, *cardiotho-racic surgeons* for heart and lungs, *colorectal surgeons* for the intestines, *neurosurgeons* for the brain, *otolaryngologists* (ear, nose, and throat doctors, or ENTs) for the head. In some situations, procedures can be done by a radiologist trained in procedures that involve imaging; these doctors are called *interventional radiologists*. If you require an operation, you will also likely meet an *anesthesiologist*, who will be responsible for putting you to sleep and keeping you out of pain during and after the surgery.

oncology, neurological surgery, ophthalmic surgery, oral and maxillofacial surgery, orthopaedic surgery, otorhinolaryngology, pediatric surgery, plastic and maxillofacial surgery, urology, vascular surgery

Other Physician Specialties

Anesthesiology, neurology, radiology, pathology

Finally, if you have had a biopsy taken during a procedure, a *pathologist* is the doctor who examines the biopsy sample to determine what it is.

Residents, Rotations, and Change of Service

Understanding the structure of who is in charge in a teaching hospital can be very difficult. In most teaching institutions, where there are residents present, it often looks like this. There is a first-year resident called the *intern*. The intern has already graduated from medical school and is technically an MD but still requires additional training before he or she can practice independently. The intern is supervised by a senior resident. In the training for the field of medicine, this might be a second- or third-year resident; however, in surgery fields with longer residencies, there will be junior residents as well. Both the intern and the resident report to the attending, who is ultimately responsible.

It is not unusual for patients to be seen by the intern first when a problem arises. Patients are most often seen by the attending during daily rounds with the team. If you want to be seen again specifically by the attending, you will have to make that clear. If you ask to be seen by the doctor, the nurse will likely send either the intern or the resident. Most teaching hospitals will also have medical students on the team. Often they introduce themselves as the student doctor. They are trained to take a medical history and do a basic physical exam. Most residents do *rotations* for about two to four weeks, the upshot being that your team may go *off service* and a new team may come *on service* while you are in the middle of your stay. The old team will pass off all your information to the new team. This can sometimes be a downside to being taken care of in a teaching hospital since it may take the new team a little extra time to learn all the details of your case. On the other hand, it is a fresh set of eyes reviewing your case, which is often beneficial.

Fellows

Another type of trainee is called a *fellow.* These physicians have finished their residency training in one medical area and have chosen to go on to more study and specialization. Some examples of fellowship training include allergy and immunology, cardiology, pulmonary and critical care, infectious disease, rheumatology, geriatrics, palliative medicine, hematology and oncology, gastroenterology, nephrology, endocrinology, and all of the surgical subspecialties, such as brain (neuro) surgery, heart surgery, etc.

Doctor's Orders

Many of us have heard the term *doctor's orders.* This refers to the instructions physicians—or in some instances, nurse practitioners or physician assistants—create to direct patient care. When physicians determine the plan of care, they will write orders for medications, tests, or physical or respiratory therapy, and these will guide your journey through the hospital. Physicians will also write orders about whether you should be in bed, move to a chair, or get up to go to the bathroom. Many of these orders are generated after consultation with the other members of the interdisciplinary health care team as well as after conversation with you and your family members. They guide the activity of a variety of other providers and health care professionals, who will in turn provide critical information to physicians about the course of your hospital stay and recovery; this information in turn will generate different orders. If, for example, a nurse notices that you do not have enough

ROUNDS

Rounds can take different forms, and the term may be confusing. If your doctor rounds in the hospital, it means that he or she is looking in on patients. The doctor may show up at any time of day or evening and might be alone. Another kind of rounds is called teaching rounds. You will see a group of medical professionals move from patient room to patient room, looking at charts and stopping at the bedside to examine patients, ultimately making decisions about care. Depending on the type of hospital, the group might be made up of student doctors, residents, fellows, nurses, physician assistants, nurse practitioners, clinical pharmacists, and attending physicians. After surgery, a team might round on the patient to make sure healing is going along properly. Typically, surgical rounds occur very early in the morning before surgeons begin their day in the operating room at about 7:30 a.m.

pain medication, she or he will alert a physician. And if that physician agrees with the nurse's assessment, he or she will order a change in medication or dose. If, for example, an order is written for pain mediation every four to six hours and you experience more frequent pain after three hours and request more medication, the nurse will locate the physician, nurse practitioner, or physician assistant to change the order. If you need to remain in a chair but wish to go to the bathroom, the nurse will locate the physician or other health care provider to request a change in the orders. These orders are the ultimate and overriding instructions. Depending on the hospital, certain orders may be telephoned in and recorded by nursing staff. Sometimes units have standing orders that do not necessitate a call to a physician, nurse practitioner, or physician assistant.

TIP   Doctor-to-Doctor Communication

You cannot assume that your doctor in the hospital will be in frequent, if any, communication with your outpatient provider. Even the most conscientious of physicians get behind on proper communication. Be sure that your inpatient provider knows the names and phone numbers of your outpatient doctors. Don't be afraid to call your outpatient doctors to tell them you are in the hospital and to provide information on who is taking care of you. Please feel empowered to ask the doctor taking care of you if he or she has spoken to and discussed the plan of care with your regular doctor. If that has not occurred, ask for the call. At a minimum, doctor-to-doctor communication should occur at the time of admission and at discharge. Communication also applies to the various doctors taking care of you in the hospital. If more than one doctor comes to see you and they tell you conflicting information, speak up and ask them to discuss things with one another. Sometimes a doctor will come to see you and will not have had a chance to speak to other doctors prior to that time. You can help communication flow between the doctors by being proactive.

PHYSICIAN HANDOFFS

There is much passing off of information between doctors. There are a couple of critical junctions where the passing of information is most important: first and foremost, admission and discharge. The attending physician must make sure to gain all necessary information from the outpatient doctor on admission. That physician must then also be sure to hand off all the information and anything requiring follow-up at the time of discharge. There are also many handoffs during the hospital stay; the day physician will sign out to the night physician, and the weekday physician will sign out to the weekend physician. Since there are so many handoffs, it is always best to try to get your questions answered by the doctor during a weekday since that doctor typically will have had more time and familiarity with your case. At other times, the covering physician may not be able to answer your questions. Be prepared that if you arrive after hours and ask to speak to the doctor, you will actually be speaking to a covering doctor. This can be frustrating, and you might not get all the information you are looking for.

TIP   Prepare Your Questions (In Other Words, Cut to the Chase)

Every doctor knows that you will have questions to ask, but your doctor has many other sick patients to care for. Be sure to maximize the time you have with your physician. Think of questions you want to ask ahead of time, and when possible write them down. Make sure you cut to the chase and get your question out.

STAYING IN TOUCH WITH YOUR DOCTOR ON THE OUTSIDE

If your own doctor has not visited or called you in the hospital, there could be several reasons for this situation. It is quite possible that he or she is not aware that you have been hospitalized if this is an unplanned admission or emergency. It is reasonable for you to call your own doctor's office to inform her or him AND the staff that you have had an inpatient admission. Or you could ask the hospital primary team physician to touch base with your doctor or doctors on the outside. We like to assume that everyone medical is communicating with everyone else. This is a bad assumption to make and can cause serious problems. Always be proactive and assume that your doctors and nurses have not been put in touch with each other. This is important at every point in your hospital stay, including shift changes and discharge.

TIP   You Can Help Ensure That All Your Providers Are Communicating with Each Other

Always be proactive and assume that your doctors and nurses have not been put in touch with each other. This is important not only at discharge but also at shift changes. You might say "Nurse, what did my specialist say when you spoke with her this morning?"

CHAPTER 7

Lines, Ports, Drains, Tubes, and Catheters

Let's face it: as a patient in the hospital you are going to get poked and prodded. If you're admitted to the hospital, chances are you will get an IV in some part of your body—usually the arms or neck. There are so many different **lines, ports, drains,** tubes, and **catheters** that can be inserted into the body. How are you supposed to know what is in you and what it is for?

A PICC Line

Bobby had had a really rough road. After he had been admitted to the hospital one week before and had many tests, the doctors had finally diagnosed him with *infective endocarditis* (a blood infection that settles in the heart). He was relieved to finally understand why he had been feeling so crummy. He was grateful to know that his illness could be treated with antibiotics. The doctor told Bobby that he would need six weeks of antibiotics through an IV. Bobby had thought, "OK, I will go home with this IV I have in my arm." The doctors had said, "Well, actually no, you will get a new special IV called a PICC line that the antibiotics can be given through." Bobby said OK. After the doctor had left the room, Bobby turned to his wife and said "Hey, what is a PICC line anyway?"

Let's take this opportunity to walk through many of the common things you might find being inserted into you as a patient in the hospital. Let's also take a moment to review Anatomy 101. You have two major types of blood vessels in your body—*arteries* and *veins*. Arteries take blood away from the heart with lots of oxygen to all the organs and tissues in the body. Veins take the blood that the organs and tissues have removed the oxygen from and bring it back to the right side of the heart. From there, the blood is sent to the lungs to get more oxygen. From the lungs it goes to the left side of the heart and back out to arteries with new oxygen. And the cycle goes on and on.

LINES

Venous Lines

Intravenous Line (IV)

An intravenous line (IV) is a small plastic tubing that is *placed* (inserted) in a *peripheral vein* (a vein in the arms, legs, hands, or feet). In order to insert an IV, a provider will place a needle in your vein. Some people are under the assumption that the needle remains in them, but this is not the case. The needle is merely a way to get into the vein. Once the vein is entered, a plastic tubing, which is mounted on the needle, is placed in the vein over the needle and the needle is removed. The IV is held in place by some kind of adhesive material, usually tape.

That's the basics. Now we will get fancy. *Lines* (sometimes also known as *catheters*) can be placed in arteries or veins and they can be located peripherally or centrally. Peripheral veins are small veins usually in the arms, legs, feet, or hands. *Central veins* are large veins in the neck, chest, or groin. The large vein in the neck most commonly used for an IV is the *internal jugular*. The large vein in the chest is either the *subclavian vein* or the *axillary vein*. The large vein in the groin is the *femoral vein*. Lines can also be tunneled or not tunneled. A *nontunneled catheter* is a fixed line that protrudes at the site of insertion. *Tunneled catheters* are inserted at one site, tunneled under the skin, and emerge at a separate site. A *port* (may also be known by its brand name *Medi-Port* or other brand names), is a tunneled catheter, but it is left completely under the skin.

There are many different kinds of lines in many different places. We will go through some of the most common you may encounter.

External Jugular (EJ) Venous IV or Catheter

The **external jugular** is a peripheral vein in the neck. This site is often chosen for a catheter when the patient needs peripheral (small vein) access but other veins cannot be accessed. It is placed in the same manner as a regular IV. The placement of this catheter has more risks than a regular IV since there is the possibility of cutting the internal jugular vein, which can lead to a significant rapid loss of blood.

Central Line (Central Venous Catheter, Central Venous Line, Central Venous Access Catheter)

The **central line** is also described by the number of channels or lumens it has—for example, single *lumen,* double *lumen*, etc. Since it is central, it is placed in one of the large veins in your neck, chest, or groin. Generally this line is placed if you have very bad veins (which means they are difficult to access) and if you need more than one medication or fluid intravenously or if your condition is **unstable** (you are very ill and at risk) and access is needed for a class of medications to increase blood pressure, known as *pressors.* The central line is put in at the bedside while you are awake. You are given some numbing medication to the skin, and the line is inserted under sterile conditions. Sometimes an *ultrasound* (see chapter 8) is used to assure proper placement. Once the line is inserted, it is sutured into place and covered with a clear adhesive material. A *chest X- ray* is often done after the procedure to ensure correct placement and to check for complications.

Peripherally Inserted Central Catheter (PICC Line)

A *peripherally inserted central catheter (PICC line)* is an intravenous line that can remain in the body for around thirty days (although in certain cases it may remain in place for months). A PICC line is used if you need prolonged antibiotics, chemotherapy, or *total parenteral nutrition (TPN,* fully explained in chapter 9). It is placed through a peripheral vein, a small vein usually in the arm, and is fed from the small vein into the larger veins until it comes to rest in the *superior vena cava* (the large vein that brings blood back to the heart). It can be placed at the bedside under sterile conditions by a trained phlebotomist or by an interventional radiologist under *fluoroscopy* (a specialized continuous X-ray).

Midline

A *midline* falls in between a regular peripheral IV and a PICC line. It is longer than a regular peripheral IV but does not pass the axillary line (in the armpit). Unlike the PICC line, it does not sit above the heart. A midline is usually placed for treatments that will be ongoing for one to six weeks. Since it is actually a type of peripheral IV, it is not appropriate for all medications. Since it is not a centrally placed line, its position and placement do not need to be confirmed with a chest X-ray.

Catheters

A catheter is a thin tube that is inserted in the body for surgery or to treat a medical condition. There are many different types of catheters, and each has a specialized purpose. They may be made of plastic, rubber, nylon, or silicon and are always made for specialized medical functions. Many lines are also referred to as catheters. And, to make matters more confusing, the terms "catheters" and "lines" may be used interchangeably.

Patient-Controlled Analgesic (PCA) Pump

A *patient-controlled analgesic (PCA) pump* is an intravenous line that is placed in a peripheral vein. Instead of being attached to fluids or antibiotics, it is attached to an electronic infusion pump. This special pump is generally filled with a strong pain medication such as a narcotic. You will be given a hand-held device with a button on the top. When you are in pain, you can self-administer another dose of pain medication by pressing the button. Many patients are initially afraid of these PCA pumps because they think that if they press the button too many times, they can overdose on pain medication. There is no need to worry, since this is not the case! The infusion pumps are electronically programmed by the medical provider to allow only a certain amount of pain medication within a certain time frame. The most common uses for these pumps in the hospital are to control pain after surgery and for cancer patients.

Arterial Lines (A-Lines)

Arterial lines are catheters placed in the artery rather than the vein; an artery is a vessel that carries blood filled with oxygen away from the heart and to the vital organs. The wrist is the most common location for placement of an A-line, but it can also be placed in the groin, inner elbow, or foot. Placement of the arterial catheter is similar to that for an IV, although the procedure is a little more involved. You will be given a medication such as *lidocaine* to numb the skin and minimize pain prior to the procedure. The catheter is *sutured*—or sewn into the skin—to hold it in place. Since the catheter is in the artery, it allows the medical providers to measure your blood pressure on a continuous basis and also to take samples of the blood without having to stick the patient again. These catheters are generally used only in the *intensive care units* (see chapter 11), where patients require continuous vital sign monitoring.

Intra-Aortic Balloon Pump (Balloon Pump or IABP)

An **intra-aortic balloon pump** is a mechanical device that, unless it is an emergency, is placed in a cardiac catheterization lab by an interventional cardiologist under fluoroscopy (a specialized continuous X-ray). It is inserted in the same manner as a central line, through the femoral vein in the leg. It is threaded from the femoral vein into the aorta and toward the heart. The most common reasons to place an IABP are to improve the blood flow through the *coronary arteries* (the blood vessels that feed the heart) and to increase *cardiac output* (blood flow out of the heart to the rest of the body).

Swan-Ganz (Pulmonary Artery) Catheter

The *Swan-Ganz catheter* is placed in the *pulmonary artery* through a central line. The pulmonary artery is the large blood vessel connecting the right ventricle of the heart to the lungs. This catheter is placed only for diagnostic purposes to get information on things such as *hemodynamics* (the flow of blood through the circulatory system). It can help the care team determine different causes of shock—for example, heart failure or *sepsis* (an overwhelming infection).

PORTS

Some patients, because of their illnesses, will need to be injected with medications for many weeks or months. In these cases, a port (a tunneled catheter that is left entirely under the skin) can be surgically implanted to aid in this process.

Medi-Port

Medi-Port is the most common brand name for a port, but there are many other patented names such as Port-a-Cath and Infuse-a-Port. A port is surgically placed under the skin and is usually seen as a bump under the skin. It is attached to a surgically placed catheter, which usually resides in a large vein such as the jugular, subclavian, or superior vena cava. The most common reasons for placement of a port are to deliver *chemotherapy* to cancer patients, total parenteral nutrition (TPN) to severely malnourished patients, blood products to patients with blood disorders, and antibiotics to patients who require a prolonged course of antibiotics. These ports are more convenient and have less risk of infection than a PICC line. They can be placed by a surgeon or interventional radiologist in an outpatient surgery setting.

Ommaya Reservoir

The *Ommaya reservoir* is a particular type of port that provides chemotherapy to the brain. It is similar to a Medi-Port but is placed under the skin of the scalp, and a catheter is threaded to the ventricle in the brain. A nurse can access this port by means of a small needle to administer chemotherapy.

DRAINS

After a surgical procedure, an interventional procedure by radiology, or a bedside procedure, a drain may be left in place. These drains allow for fluid drainage that may continue after the procedure has taken place. Drains can exit from any anatomical location in your body. The most common areas to find drains are from the head, the chest cavity (near heart and lungs), the abdominal cavity (near digestive organs), and the extremities (arms and legs). The nurse taking care of you will often empty these drains of their contents and record the amount of fluid to determine if and when the drain can be removed.

The *Jackson-Pratt (JP) drain* is one type of drainage device that works on a suction mechanism. The drain (a thin plastic tube) is left in place after a surgical procedure, with the end of the drain connected to a plastic bulb. When a member of the health care team removes the plug from the end of the bulb, squeezes the air out, and replaces the bulb, suction is created. Typically, the nurse will drain the contents of the bulb and record the amount of fluid that was inside to determine with the other providers when removal is appropriate.

Drains to Remove Fluids

Dennis couldn't believe he was only forty-eight years old and stuck in the hospital. His right side had been bothering him for over a week. It wasn't until he developed a fever that his wife had dragged him into the emergency room. The doctors told him he had an abscess in one of his muscles and would have to undergo a procedure to drain it. Fast-forward to one day later: Dennis had had the procedure to drain the abscess—needless to say, he was shocked to find a tube sticking out of his side when he returned to his room. No less, the tube had a funny-looking plastic bulb on the end of it that was collecting some kind of fluid.

TUBES

Oxygen (O$_2$)

Oxygen is essential to sustain life. Even if it is not really needed, many patients feel comforted just by having supplemental oxygen. The most common way to receive oxygen in the hospital is by something called a *nasal cannula,* plastic tubing with two short tubes sticking out that rest in your nostrils. The tubing is held in place by wrapping it behind your ears and is attached usually to an oxygen valve in the wall at the bedside.

The tubing can also be attached to a portable oxygen tank if you leave the room for a test or a procedure. The nurse can check how the oxygen level is doing by putting a plastic clip on the finger called a *pulse oximeter.* If this level of oxygen is insufficient to improve the level of oxygen in the blood, the nurse or doctor may attach the oxygen tubing to a mask that goes over your nose and mouth. Higher levels of oxygen are able to be given this way.

Endotracheal (ET or Breathing) Tube

The *endotracheal tube* is probably the most frightening type of tube you will see in the hospital. This tube is inserted down your *trachea* (windpipe) when you are having difficulty breathing. These breathing tubes can then be hooked up to a ventilator (respirator), which will breathe for you when you cannot breathe for yourself.

Chest Tubes

The chest cavity is very complex. Working from the outside in there are skin, fat, muscle, bone, and lungs. The lungs are covered by a tissue called *pleura*, which also covers the inside of the ribs. There is a small space between the two layers of pleura called the *pleural space.* If air gets into that space, the lung can collapse; this is called a *pneumothorax.* If fluid gets into that space, it is called a *pleural effusion.* If pus gets into that space, it is called an *empyema.* A *chest tube* is a small plastic tube that is placed through the side of the chest into the pleural space. This allows for drainage of whatever is in the pleural space. Often the chest tube is hooked up to a box that has a series of chambers in it. This box allows for the drainage of fluid and makes sure there are no air leaks in the system. Chest tubes are usually placed at the bedside under sterile conditions, after the skin is numbed, by doctors, nurse practitioners, or physician assistants who have received special training to perform this procedure.

Percutaneous Gastrostomy (PEG) Tube

Also known as a *feeding tube,* the *percutaneous gastrostomy (PEG) tube* is placed either for patients who are unable to eat because of swallowing difficulties (*dysphagia*) or for patients who need additional nutrition. A small flexible tube is placed into your stomach from the skin overlying the stomach. A bumper is inflated inside your stomach so the tube cannot fall out. Once this tube is in place, you can receive liquid nutrition either continuously or in a *bolused* (all at once) fashion. When the tube is passed from the stomach into the second part of the small intestine called the *jejunum*, it is called a *jejunostomy tube* or *J tube*. This tube can be placed by a gastroenterologist, an interventional radiologist, or a surgeon.

Nasogastric (NG) Tube (NGT)

The *nasogastric (NG) tube* is placed down your nose through the esophagus and into your stomach and allows for feeding and medication administration if you are unable to swallow or eat for a variety of medical reasons. It can come in different sizes depending on what the indication for the tube is. It is temporary and cannot stay in for more than two weeks.

Nephrostomy Tube

The *nephrostomy tube* is a kidney tube (*nephro* pertains to the kidney). Normally the kidney makes urine and the urine passes out of the kidneys, down the *ureter*, into the *bladder*, down the *urethra*, and out of the body. If there is a block somewhere in this system, the urine is unable to get out. To release pressure in the system and to prevent kidney injury, a nephrostomy tube can be placed. This is a small plastic tube that is passed from the skin to a part of your kidney. Bags are attached to the tubes to collect the urine. Either an interventional radiologist or a surgeon can perform this procedure.

URINARY CATHETERS

The *urinary (Foley) catheter* is flexible tubing that is placed into your bladder to collect urine. This catheter is placed at the bedside under sterile conditions for both men and women. A balloon is inflated at the end inside the bladder so that it does not fall out. The catheter is attached to a bag that collects the urine and is often hung at the bedside. If you need to leave the hospital with a Foley still in place, you will be given a smaller bag that is held to your leg via an elastic band.

CHAPTER 8

Tests and Procedures in the Hospital

Just as most people do not make it through their hospital experience without having an IV placed (inserted), most also end up having to undergo at least one test or a procedure. This chapter will explain different kinds of tests you might get while being a patient in the hospital. The first section is a description of tests that may apply for many different illnesses and for many different body parts. The rest of the chapter is broken down by the different specialties under which these tests are generally ordered or performed. The descriptions are given for a basic understanding—if you have learned that you will undergo one of these procedures and have further questions, you should ask the doctors and nurses caring for you.

TIP Diagnostic Uncertainty

Not being sure of what your actual diagnosis is can lead physicians to order many tests to help determine the diagnosis. Not all these tests are always necessary. In addition, there may be other less expensive or less invasive ways to ascertain a diagnosis. You should always feel empowered to ask your doctor what test you are having and what the *indication* (reason) for the test is.

VITAL SIGNS: TEMPERATURE, BLOOD PRESSURE, HEART RATE, AND PULSE OXIMETRY

This group of simple tests to check your vital signs will be performed repeatedly during your hospital stay. In fact, you as a patient will probably adapt to the routine of nurses who come into your room at regular intervals to administer these tests. The interval will depend on the reason for your admission and your condition, usually ranging between four and eight hours. Unfortunately, because of patient safety concerns, patients may often be woken up so clinicians can gain important information from these tests. Your temperature will be taken by mouth to see if there is a fever, a blood pressure cuff will be wrapped around your arm, and the nurse will listen with a stethoscope to hear your blood pressure. Your wrist pulse may also be taken. *Pulse oximetry* will be done on your finger to see if the blood is getting enough oxygen. As you may imagine, a large change in any reading on these basic tests may signal to the nurse that your condition is worsening. Therefore, please understand that even when you may be resting, it is for your safety that the nurse obtains the information from these tests.

BLOOD TESTS (BLOOD WORK)

There is much information about the general state of health provided by the blood: infection, heart function (cardiac enzymes), anemia, liver problems, and elevated sugars are just a few of the conditions that can be diagnosed from the blood. Therefore, blood tests are a routine diagnostic step to gather information about what brought you to the hospital or to monitor your condition. If a certain illness is suspected, the tests might be very specific. Other sets of blood tests cast a wide net when the diagnosis is not obvious. Some blood results can be seen immediately, while others take hours, even days, to be determined. Rest assured that treatment is never delayed in serious situations while your providers are waiting for blood work results.

Following are some common blood tests you are likely to have done.

CBC (Complete Blood Count)

A *CBC (complete blood count)* will show your *hemoglobin, hematocrit, white blood cell count,* and *platelet count.* Hemoglobin and hematocrit will reveal whether you are *anemic* (low in red blood cells that carry oxygen throughout the body). There are many reasons why someone might be anemic, so this finding would be a starting point for more tests. A low hemoglobin and hematocrit reading may also be indicative of bleeding somewhere in your body. *Internal bleeds* (bleeding that is not visible), if severe, can be quite dangerous. The white blood cell count can expose an infection. The platelet count reveals how well your blood will clot if you bleed.

Chemistry

The *chemistry,* also known as the *basic metabolic panel,* looks at such things as *sodium, potassium, blood urea nitrogen (BUN), creatinine,* and *glucose* levels. The *sodium level* indicates the level of hydration, potassium is an electrolyte important for proper cardiac (heart) function, the BUN and creatinine indicate kidney function, and glucose is blood sugar.

Triglycerides and Cholesterol and Liver Function Tests

Tests for *triglycerides* and *cholesterol* reveal the level of fat and cholesterol in the blood. Liver function tests, which measure *transaminases* (liver enzymes), may be performed to test for liver damage.

Sedimentation Rate and C Reactive Protein (CRP)

Sedimentation rate and *C reactive protein (CRP)* are blood tests that assess the level of inflammation in the body.

Hemoglobin A1C

Hemoglobin A1C is a blood test common to diabetics that is able to measure the level of glucose control over the past three months by looking at the amount of glucose on red blood cells.

Coagulation Profile

A *coagulation profile* is a test that tells how thin your blood is and is important when you are on the blood thinners *heparin* and *warfarin*

(*Coumadin* is the brand name). You may hear the terms *INR/PT (international normalized ratio/prothrombin time)* and *PTT(partial thromboplastin time)* referring to this type of blood test. INR/PT and PTT are the blood tests that reveal how thin your blood is by timing how long it takes the blood to clot.

GENERAL IMAGING TESTS

TIP   A Word about Medical Language

You may hear the health professionals refer to your test as a "study." This does not mean you will be part of a study or will have to read up to take an exam. In this context, a study means a test. You will also hear certain types of radiology tests referred to as "imaging" since the radiologist will obtain a picture.

Radiograph (X-ray)

X-rays are done for many different reasons and are one of the most common diagnostic tools. If you are suspected of having a broken bone, you will undergo an X-ray *(radiograph)* evaluation. It is standard policy in many hospitals for all adult patients being admitted to undergo a *baseline* (the first version of a test, against which subsequent versions will be compared) chest X-ray. If you have severe abdominal pain, you may undergo an X-ray to look for a blockage. The hospital worker who administers an X-ray is called a radiology technician (or "tech" for short). You might be able to remain in your room or cubicle for this test if portable X-ray machines are available. If not, you will be transported to an X-ray room, where you will be given a heavy shield made of lead to protect the parts of your body that do not require imaging. You may be asked to lie down, sit, or stand, depending on the type of X-ray needed and the part of the body under investigation. X-rays use radiation to look inside the body; this is an extremely useful source of medical information. However, we now know that radiation, and by extension, too many X-rays, may be harmful to human tissue. There are many other sources of radiation that we are exposed to in the environment, and we do not discourage the use of X-rays. However, it is entirely appropriate to ask the doctors and nurses if an X-ray is necessary to make the diagnosis.

Computed Tomography (CT) or Computed Axial Tomography (CAT) Scan

A *CT (also called CAT) scan* is useful as a way to see what an X-ray cannot see. Where an X-ray can usually determine if there is a broken bone, a CT scan can peer inside to the internal organs. If you came to the hospital with trouble breathing, a CT scan of the lungs may be the best method to see pneumonia, fluid in the lungs, or a *pulmonary embolism* (blood clot in the lungs). If you came to the hospital with abdominal pain, a CT scan may be the best way to see a blockage in the intestines or an inflammation or infection such as *colitis* (infection or inflammation of the large bowel). Depending on the reason for your CT scan, the health care provider may ask you to drink large quantities of a flavored liquid. This substance is a contrast material that helps to differentiate the organs to be viewed. The type of CT scan will be determined on the basis of the symptoms, the illness suspected, and the safety of the test for each individual. If there is a problem with the kidneys, a CT might not be a suitable test if it is done with IV contrast. The decision about the appropriate test will be made after weighing all the pros and cons. Since CTs are made of many (hundreds) X-rays, there has been concern about exposure to too much radiation. There have been tremendous improvements in reducing the amount of radiation for certain CT equipment; however, not all hospitals have acquired these newer machines. If you have had repeated CTs in the past, you may want to discuss with the doctor whether another technology form can be substituted. You may also want to ask about the age and quality of the equipment your hospital uses.

Magnetic Resonance Imaging (MRI)

While CT scans are suited for bone injuries, lung and chest imaging, and cancer detection, an *MRI* is better suited for tendon and ligament problems, spinal cord issues, and brain tumors. An MRI does not have the radiation exposure of a CT scan. Unfortunately, it usually takes about thirty minutes to perform, whereas a CT scan takes five minutes. In addition, many hospitals do not have open MRI equipment, and some patients find the closed MRI setup makes them feel claustrophobic, since you are placed on a narrow board and your body is put through an imaging machine in a confined space. You will not be able to have an MRI if you have had metal inserted in your body—for example, older pacemakers and metal rods for orthopaedic procedures. For your safety, you will be asked to fill out a questionnaire prior to going for the MRI.

SPECIALTY-SPECIFIC TESTS

Cardiology

Stress Testing

Stress tests are often conducted in the outpatient setting as a routine part of diagnosis by cardiologists. If you are admitted for chest pain, depending on your risk factors, you will have several tests to see if you have any blockages in the coronary arteries (the arteries that supply blood to the heart). There are many different types of stress tests; the one best suited to your condition will be selected. The stress test assesses the heart's ability to perform when it is being challenged in some way, often by strenuous exercise. The test will push your heart to its limits to reveal if there are rhythm abnormalities or insufficient blood flow. This can be accomplished two different ways. Either you will be asked to walk on a treadmill at increasing inclines and increasing speeds or you will be given an injection of a medication that will speed up your heart. An EKG (*electrocardiogram*) will be taken while you are exercising (*exercise stress test*); in the other type of stress test you are given an injection of a *radiotracer* that allows pictures of your heart to be taken (*nuclear stress test*). Another type of stress test involves an *echocardiogram* (ultrasound of the heart) that is taken before and after the exercise portion of the test (*stress echocardiography*). To ensure your safety, stress tests are administered under the watchful eyes of physicians and trained technicians.

Cardiac Catheterization

Cardiac catheterization includes the X-ray portion of the test, which is called an *angiogram*. In cardiac catheterization, a thin tube is inserted into the blood vessels. This is an *invasive* (through the skin or into the body) test that allows visualization of the blood flow through the coronary arteries; cardiac catheterization also can be used to open up any blockages. This test is performed if you appear to have certain types of acute heart attacks or abnormal findings on a stress test. This test can also be useful to evaluate the valves and pressures in your heart. You will be awake for the procedure. An IV will be placed in either your groin or your wrist. The doctor will inject a contrast dye, and continuous pictures will be taken with a *fluoroscopy* machine (which provides live X-ray pictures) to see if there are defects or areas of blockage. If there are blockages, you may have an *angioplasty* (in which a balloon pushes open the blockage) or possibly have a *stent* placed, which holds the artery open.

Echocardiography

Echocardiography involves a sonogram of the heart and is performed the same way as a sonogram procedure for any other part of the body. An *ultrasound* technician or a cardiologist will place sonogram jelly on your chest and will use a probe to obtain images of the heart. The test allows the cardiologist to see the structure of the heart, including the walls, the valves, and the blood flow across these structures. When the echo is done this way, it is called a *transthoracic echo (TTE)*. Sometimes the doctor may need to get a better look at a part of your heart that sits farther toward the back. If this is the case, you might need a special echocardiogram called a *transesophageal echo (TEE)*. You are usually given some type of sedating medication for this procedure since a scope is placed down your throat into your esophagus (food pipe).

Electrophysiology (EP) Testing and Ablation

The heart can beat too fast or too slowly, or it can have a regular rhythm or an irregular rhythm. A cardiologist who specializes in heart rhythms, a *cardiac electrophysiologist*, performs specific tests to figure out the source of the rhythm problem. *Electrophysiology testing* (also known as *EP testing* or *study*) is done in a fashion very similar to that for the cardiac catheterization described above. The difference is that electrode catheters are threaded up to your heart to record electrical signals and, when necessary, can *ablate* (remove tissue from) the area of the heart that is sending out bad signals.

Automatic Implantable Cardioverter Defibrillator (AICD) and Permanent Pacemaker (PPM)

Sometimes, depending on your heart problems, you are at risk for sudden cardiac arrest; this means that your heart stops beating. If your doctor feels you are at risk for this condition, it is possible to have an *automatic implantable cardioverter defibrillator (AICD)* implanted in your heart. This device senses the heart rhythm and can shock your heart out of a dangerous rhythm or shock you if your heart stops. Sometimes your heart does not beat as quickly as it should or does not beat properly because of an electrical problem. If this is the case, you can have a *permanent pacemaker (PPM)* implanted, which can regulate your heart rate. Both devices are placed by a simple surgical procedure for which you are given a sedative.

Cardioversion

If your heart is going too fast or your heart rhythm is too irregular and it becomes difficult to maintain blood pressure, the doctor will shock you—a procedure known as *cardioversion.* This is done by placing sticky pads attached to a *defibrillator* (a machine that can deliver an electric shock) to your chest. This is done in a controlled environment, and a light sedative is usually given. Your doctor will work with a team of other health care professionals to provide the best outcome for your cardioversion. Other members of the health care team may include a nurse, nurse practitioner, physician assistant, cardiology technician, X-ray technician, anesthesiologist, and pharmacist.

Tilt Table

If you have come to the hospital with complaints of dizziness or have passed out, changes in your position may be affecting your blood pressure and heart rate. In this situation, a *tilt table* test might be ordered. During this test, you will be strapped down to a flat table and instructed not to move. Your blood pressure and heart rate are monitored as the table is slowly tilted into an upright position. The doctor and technicians can determine if there has been a significant drop in your blood pressure or rise in your heart rate that may have caused the symptoms.

Many Tests to Figure Out a Cardiac Problem

Frank knew he was getting old—he would be almost eighty this year. He had managed to stay out of doctors' offices and hospitals almost his whole life. But now look where he had landed! He was in a hospital bed, on a cardiology floor, no less, with wires and other stuff hooked up to him. He wasn't expecting to be there. In fact, he had been at his granddaughter's wedding, and everything had been going just fine until she was just about to say "I do." He had started to feel sweaty, and the next thing he knew he was on the floor with people hovering over him and telling him the ambulance was on its way. Well, now he was stuck in the hospital—the doctor had just told him he would need to have some tests to figure out why he had passed out. Something about an echocardiogram, stress test, and tilt table test.

Dermatology: Skin Biopsy

A rash can be completely benign or can be a sign of something more serious; often the only way to tell is through a *skin biopsy.* This is generally a simple procedure that the dermatologist can do at your bedside with a little locally injected pain medication. After injection of the medication, usually *lidocaine,* in the area, the doctor will use a *scalpel* (surgical knife) to cut off a small sample.

Endocrinology

ACTH Stimulation Test (Cosyntropin Test)

As a result of the media attention steroids receive, when people hear about them, most think of big, bulky bodybuilders and athletes. Those are people who inject themselves with steroids they are not supposed to use. The body makes its own natural steroids, which are important for many critical body functions, including maintaining normal blood pressure. Two glands sitting on top of each of your kidneys, called *adrenal glands,* are responsible for making these steroids. If your doctor suspects that your adrenal glands are not making the steroids properly—a condition called *adrenal insufficiency*—he or she may order an **ACTH stimulation test.** **ACTH** is a substance normally found in your pituitary gland that tells your adrenal glands to make steroids. You will have a blood test done before the test to check your steroid level, and the steroid being tested is **cortisol.** Then, somewhere between thirty and sixty minutes after injection with the ACTH, your blood will be checked again to see whether the cortisol level has increased. The results of this test will allow the doctor to see whether your pituitary and adrenal glands are functioning normally.

Thyroid Scan

The thyroid is a gland that resides in your neck; it controls the **metabolism** through several types of **hormones** (substances that control functions and activities in the body). Think of it as a car engine; sometimes it goes into overdrive (**hyperthyroidism**) and sometimes it runs out of gas (**hypothyroidism**). A **thyroid scan** uses radioactivity and takes pictures to determine the areas in your thyroid that may be overactive or underactive. It can also be used to evaluate nodules to help determine if they are benign or malignant (cancerous).

Gastroenterology

Abdominal Ultrasound

Ultrasound provides a picture of the insides of your body. An **abdominal ultrasound** can look at many organs, but most often, this test will be used to look at your liver, the ducts that run through it, as well as your gallbladder, spleen, kidneys, and bladder. It is a common test given when you complain of abdominal pain, particularly when the pain occurs on your upper right-hand side, indicating a problem with the gallbladder, such as an infection due to a stone blocking the gallbladder from draining. An abdominal ultrasound is an excellent noninvasive way to look for an infected gallbladder.

Colonoscopy

A **colonoscopy** allows a good look inside the colon, which is the large intestine. There may be many different reasons why your health care provider would want to look in your colon. Colonoscopies are a standard screening test for colon cancer and are often performed in an outpatient setting.

When patients come into the hospital for abdominal pain, tender bellies, or inability to keep food down, the colonoscopy is useful to look for sources of bleeding, infection, or inflammation. Since the gastroenterologist will want a nice clean colon to drive the scope through to see all there is to see, you will need to take some sort of laxative preparation the day before the procedure. Different hospitals have different "prep" protocols, which can range from a combination of pills to enemas to liquid drinks. The procedure is done under light sedation in the endoscopy suite by the gastroenterologist. A scope is passed from your rectum throughout the entirety of the colon.

TIP   Prepping for a Colonoscopy

If you are being prepped in the hospital for a colonoscopy and you are not in a private room or in the bed by the bathroom, you might want to consider requesting a portable commode for convenience as you will likely have to move your bowels many times during the night.

Esophagogastroduodenoscopy (EGD)
An *esophagogastroduodenoscopy (EGD)* allows a look at the upper part of the gastrointestinal tract and does not require any special preparation except that you can't have anything to eat or drink six hours prior to the procedure. Patients will be given a light sedative in the endoscopy suite of the hospital. The gastroenterologist will place a scope in your throat, down your esophagus, and into your stomach. This allows the health care team to see if there is anything wrong in the esophagus, stomach, and uppermost part of the small intestine (duodenum). If there is evidence of something concerning, a *biopsy* (removing a piece of tissue for evaluation by a *pathologist*) may be performed. Likewise, during the procedure, if bleeding is noted, attempts will be made to stop it.

Lots of Ways to Look at the Intestines

My husband relayed a funny story once in which he heard older men in the locker room at the gym saying they had to go to the gastroenterologist for an "around the world." Later I came to realize this meant an EGD and colonoscopy—a look into the gastrointestinal tract from above and below.—*Karen Friedman*

Endoscopic Retrograde Cholangiopancreatography (ERCP)

You will see that the EGD, described above, gets to the first part of your small intestine. The **endoscopic retrograde cholangiopancreatography (ERCP)** is performed in the same fashion as the EGD, but once the scope is inside the first part of the small bowel (the duodenum), dye can be injected into the ductal system that connects to the liver/gallbladder and pancreas. The doctor and technicians use fluoroscopy (live X-rays) to see if there is anything going wrong within the system. This test can be diagnostic—they are merely trying to figure out what the problem is. Or it can be therapeutic—meaning they may try to remove a blocked stone or place a stent to open up a closed-off area. Just like the EGD, the ERCP is done with a light sedative in a radiology suite.

Endoscopic Ultrasound

Also known as **EUS**, the **endoscopic ultrasound** combines an endoscopy (a scope down a hollow organ) with an ultrasound, which allows visualization of adjacent organs more easily. If necessary, a biopsy may be performed during this procedure. If a gastroenterologist is doing this procedure, there will be a combination of the EGD (described above) with an ultrasound component. If a pulmonologist (lung doctor) is doing this procedure, the ultrasound can be combined with a **bronchoscopy.**

Capsule Endoscopy

The EGD gets the scope down to the first part of your small bowel. The colonoscopy gets a look at your entire colon. What about the part of the small bowel left in between? There is a good way for a gastroenterologist to visualize this stretch of bowel. A **capsule endoscopy** is performed with a pill-sized camera that you swallow. As the camera travels through the digestive tract, it takes pictures that are transmitted to an external recording device you wear. The pictures can be uploaded to a computer and interpreted by a gastroenterologist. If you are to undergo capsule endoscopy, you will likely be a given a laxative the day before the procedure to clear the digestive tract.

Nasogastric Tube (NGT)

A *nasogastric tube* (NGT) is a flexible plastic tube that can be inserted in your nostril and is passed down the back of your throat, down your esophagus, and into your stomach. The insertion procedure is done at the bedside, usually with some anesthetic medication to your nostril and the back of your throat. It is important that you make sure you get an anesthetic for the insertion. While it is uncomfortable to have it inserted, it is usually well tolerated once in place. After insertion, a chest X-ray is done to confirm proper placement. There are several reasons why you may need to have an NGT inserted. If there is some kind of obstruction in your bowel, its contents may need to be removed with a suction canister hooked up to the NGT. If you have difficulty swallowing (dysphagia) or are at risk for aspiration, food and medications can be delivered via the NGT directly into your stomach. Liquid food, liquid medications, and crushed pills can be placed down the NGT.

TIP   NG Tube Placement and Removal

Placement (insertion) of the NG tube is uncomfortable, but most likely you will adjust to it after a short period. You may also find the removal of the tube uncomfortable. Our advice is to ask the doctor to pull it out fairly quickly.

Paracentesis

Sometimes there is fluid in your abdomen that is not supposed to be there. Your health care provider may know why the fluid is there or may be trying to figure the reason why this is so. *Paracentesis* is a procedure to remove fluid from the abdomen. If the amount removed is small, this is a diagnostic paracentesis. This small sample can be analyzed to reveal the reason for the presence of fluid. If there is a substantial amount of fluid in the abdomen causing discomfort, a larger amount will be removed; this is called a therapeutic paracentesis. These procedures can be done at the bedside by most trained physicians. The procedure is done in a sterile fashion to prevent infection. You will be given a local anesthetic at the area on your abdomen where the needle will go in. A diagnostic paracentesis procedure takes only a few moments, whereas a therapeutic procedure paracentesis will take longer, depending on the amount of fluid that is removed.

Rectal Tube
Sometimes the amount of diarrhea a patient has is uncontrollable. In certain instances a doctor may place plastic tubing called a *rectal tube* into the rectum. This tube is connected to a bag that will collect the stool. This intervention will not stop the diarrhea but will help limit soiling, which can be harmful to the skin or may increase risk of infection. Rectal tubes are also a method of relieving gas in some patients who have trouble passing gas after surgery.

Geriatrics

Cognitive Testing
Many patients come to the hospital with confusion from dementia, and others may become confused while in the hospital—a condition known as *delirium*. Doctors and nurses will often try to determine a patient's mental ability through *cognitive testing* with the *mini mental status exam (MMSE)*. This is a thirty-point questionnaire revolving around questions of orientation and specific cognitive skills. A high score denotes high-level mental status, while a low score signals dementia.

Confusion Assessment Method (CAM)
Many patients, particularly the elderly, are at risk for *delirium* during a hospital stay. Patients with dementia at baseline are at higher risk for delirium. Additionally, serious illness, injury, and anesthesia may tip you into delirium. Nurses and physicians use the *confusion assessment method (CAM)* to check patients for confusion to prevent episodes of delirium. The CAM consists of several questions that may be asked at the bedside.

Gynecology (Women's Reproductive Health)

Pelvic Exam
A *pelvic exam* is done so the doctor or other health care professional can look at the cervix and take swab samples to look for infections that could be causing the symptoms.

Pelvic Ultrasound

Even though CT scans can generally see well into your body and your pelvic area, sometimes a *pelvic ultrasound* can gather more useful information. This is considered a noninvasive procedure. It is performed with an ultrasound probe over the abdomen and an additional probe placed in the vagina. (Note that men requiring pelvic ultrasound will have the probe inserted in the rectum.) These procedures are done either by a radiologist, ultrasound technician, or gynecologist. There is mild discomfort, and the procedure usually takes only a few minutes.

Hematology/Oncology

Bone Marrow Biopsy

Bone marrow is responsible for making many different kinds of blood cells such as red blood cells and platelets. When blood tests reveal that one or all of the major cell lines are decreased, such as in *anemia* (decreased red blood cells), or even increased, you may need a *bone marrow biopsy* to determine the cause. This procedure is done at the bedside. Usually the biopsy is done on the hip bone. Your hip will be injected with lidocaine (an anesthetic to decrease pain) and then a large needle is inserted down into your hip bone to obtain a sample. While the procedure can be painful for some, most people complain only of feeling pressure.

Transfusions

If the blood tests reveal that you are *anemic*, it means that your body does not have enough red blood cells. Red blood cells are responsible for carrying oxygen to all the tissues in your body. If you are severely anemic, you will require a *transfusion* of red blood cells. You will need a blood test prior to transfusion to determine your blood type to decrease the risk of a reaction; this is called a *type and screen*. It will take about three hours to transfuse an entire bag of blood. The transfusion is run through the intravenous line and does not cause discomfort. Another common type of transfusion is for *platelets*. Platelets are blood cells that help in the clotting process. A platelet transfusion does not require a type and screen prior to infusion since the platelets are not blood type-dependent. Platelet transfusions are pooled from many different donors.

TIP   Risks and Benefits of Red Blood Cell Transfusions

Red blood cell transfusions have risks and benefits, which should be explained to you prior to your signing a consent form. Some complications include infection and allergic reaction. The timing of a complication ranges from immediately up to several years. If an explanation is not offered to you, be sure to ask your health care providers to go over these risks and how your individual situation affects the possible benefits and potential downside.

Radiation Therapy

Radiation is most commonly a form of treatment for cancer, although it can be used to treat other medical conditions as well. *Radiation therapy* damages cancer cells, preventing them from growing. Sometimes radiation therapy is the only treatment, and sometimes it is combined with other treatments such as surgery or *chemotherapy* (medication to treat cancer or other diseases). Radiation is given by a specialist doctor called a radiation oncologist and is administered in a specialized area in the hospital. Often, the treatment requires you to lie flat for a period of time. The radiation beams are aimed specifically to avoid exposing any of the healthy parts of your body. Before undergoing treatment, you will be *mapped,* in a process by which the radiation oncologist determines exactly where the beams will be directed and how many treatments of radiation are needed. For safety, there is a lifetime limit to the amount of radiation you should receive, so a very precise mathematical calculation will occur.

Nephrology

Twenty-Four-Hour Urine Testing

Twenty-four-hour urine testing is easy to administer and easy for you to undergo. It is most commonly used to determine how much protein is in your urine. The nurse will place a large plastic container in your room in which all your urine is collected over a twenty-four-hour period and then sent to the laboratory. If you have been asked to do this test, make sure not to urinate in the toilet and flush it by mistake. You will likely be asked to urinate into a plastic "hat" placed over your toilet seat or into a plastic urinal if you are a male. The nurse will then empty the hats into the twenty-four-hour container. If you flush your urine by accident, be sure to tell the nurse.

Dialysis

We cannot do justice to *dialysis* in one paragraph; countless textbooks have been written about the subject. The important points to know are that sometimes your kidneys can fail for many different reasons. When this happens, you lose the ability to get rid of toxins and to balance certain *electrolytes* (naturally occurring minerals in the body) such as potassium. Dialysis—either *hemo* (filtering the blood) or *peritoneal* (filtering through the liquid made in the abdominal cavity that surrounds the organs) is a way to get rid of toxins and balance electrolytes for your failing kidneys. The most common type of dialysis in the hospital is hemodialysis, and this is done through a large intravenous line called a Shiley, which is placed in either your groin or your neck. If you are on dialysis, you will have blood work monitored daily.

Neurology

Lumbar Puncture

Lumbar puncture is a procedure in which a needle is inserted into your spinal canal to extract some fluid for analysis. It is useful to diagnose certain conditions such as meningitis and other infections of the central nervous system or brain. It has a reputation (which it has lived up to) for causing some discomfort, possibly pain, and it sometimes results in headaches after the procedure. A lumbar puncture can be performed by ER attending doctors, internists, and neurologists. While you are either lying on your side or sitting up and leaning over, your lower back will be injected with lidocaine to numb the area. Then a needle will be inserted through the space between your back bones to extract a sample of fluid. This fluid is then sent to the lab to determine if there is an infection and whether it is bacterial, viral, or caused by parasites.

Speech and Swallow Testing

Older patients with decreased mental status may have difficulty swallowing. It is also possible to develop a swallowing problem while in the hospital as the result of an invasive procedure, such as mechanical ventilation.

If you cannot swallow safely, you are at risk of *aspiration*, a process whereby the food can land in the lungs instead of the stomach, which can lead to pneumonia. A speech and swallow therapist may be called in for a consultation. The first step will be a bedside exam in which you will be given some food and drink to assess the integrity of the swallowing mechanism. If you do not do well during this exam, you may need further swallow testing such as *barium swallow*. In this test, you will drink a liquid containing *barium* (a radiopaque substance that can be seen on X-ray). X-rays will be taken while you swallow to determine the cause of the swallowing problem.

Orthopaedics: Joint Aspiration

These days many patients have their joints (knees, shoulders, and hips) replaced with artificial *implants*. Occasionally these new joints get infected. Patients turn up at the hospital in pain, with fevers, swelling, and stiffness. If the orthopaedist suspects an infection, you may have a needle inserted into the joint to extract some fluid for testing (*joint aspiration*). If the test shows an infection, you will be admitted for IV antibiotics to prepare for another surgery.

Plastic Surgery: Debridement

Debridement is the removal of dead tissue. It is often necessary to remove dead tissue and surrounding infected tissue so that your healthy tissue can survive. There are many different types of debridement, but a common one is done at your bedside by a surgeon, a dermatologist, or a nurse who is a wound-care specialist. As the top dead layer of skin is often devoid of nerves, this is often done without anesthetic. A *scalpel* (surgical knife) is used to cut back the dead skin and expose the underlying healthy skin so it can flourish.

Pulmonology

Thoracentesis
Sometimes there is fluid in the space surrounding your lungs that is not supposed to be there. It may be that your doctor already knows why the

fluid is there, or he or she may still be trying to figure it out. A *thoracentesis* is a procedure to remove that fluid; the amount may be small or large or somewhere in between. The pulmonary doctor can look at a small sample and try to figure out what is causing the problem. This procedure can be done at the bedside by most trained physicians, either a resident or an attending. (Hospitals have protocols to determine who is qualified to do the procedure.) You will be given a local anesthetic to numb the area on your chest wall where the needle will be inserted, and the procedure is done in a sterile fashion. The length of the procedure will depend on how much fluid is in the space surrounding the lungs.

Bronchoscopy

Just as an endoscopy looks into the stomach and a colonoscopy looks into your colon, a **bronchoscopy** allows a look into your lungs. There are many different reasons for a bronchoscopy. Sometimes it is necessary to get a fluid or tissue sample to determine what kind of infection is present or if there is a cancer present. The procedure is done in a bronchoscopy suite with an interdisciplinary team. Members of the team often include a nurse, an anesthesiologist, a bronchoscopy technician, and a pulmonary doctor. You will be given a sedative medication so you are not awake for the procedure. The doctor will put the scope down your throat, into your trachea (windpipe), and down into the bronchus (large airway), so that pictures can be taken as well as samples of the tissue. During the procedure, the large airways can be cleared out if necessary.

Ventilation/Perfusion (VQ) Scan

A *pulmonary embolism* (PE), which is also known as a *pulmonary embolus,* is a blood clot that has traveled through the veins and gotten lodged in the lungs. It is another condition your health care team will be concerned about if you come to the hospital short of breath. To diagnose a PE, the two main choices of tests are a CT scan with contrast or a *ventilation/perfusion (V/Q) scan.* If there is a reason, such as abnormal kidney function, that the CT scan is not suitable, you will have a V/Q scan. For this procedure you will be asked to inhale an aerosolized radioactive material through a mouthpiece, and then you will be scanned by a special camera. Through the inhaled radioactive material, the doctor and technicians can see by pictures if there are mismatches in areas of your lung between the air coming in (*ventilation*) and the blood flow (*perfusion*). Areas with a large mismatch might mean you have a PE. Radiation exposure in this test is considered low.

Rheumatology: Arthrocentesis

Your joints can collect fluid that can be from an infection or from blood if there has been recent trauma. Sometimes there might be crystals present, as in the case of gout. An *arthrocentesis* is a procedure used to remove and then examine the fluid. This test is done at your bedside. To numb the area, you will be injected with lidocaine, an anesthetic to reduce pain. A large needle will be inserted to remove a fluid sample. The procedure is generally well tolerated (not too much pain).

General Surgery: Incision and Drainage

The *incision and drainage* procedure is exactly like it sounds: the doctor cuts something open and lets the stuff inside drain out. A surgeon may find an infected area under your skin. You can think of it as a giant pimple. Antibiotics have a hard time getting inside a walled-off site of infection, so the best way to help cure the infection is to let it drain out. The doctor will inject your skin with a numbing medication first and then use a scalpel (surgical knife) to open the area. Afterward the site is covered with a *dressing* (sterile bandage).

Urology

Urinary Catheter (Foley) Placement

This is probably one of the most common procedures done in the hospital, second only to IV insertion. A Foley catheter is a plastic tube that is inserted in your urethra to help drain the urine from the bladder. There are many different reasons for a Foley placement, ranging from your inability to *void* (urinate) properly, too much blood in the urine, or the need to get a very accurate measurement of urine output. The procedure is done at your bedside usually by the nurse, and it takes only a few moments. The procedure may cause some discomfort, but once the tube is in, you probably will quickly forget that it is there. Nurses, nurse practitioners, physician assistants, and physicians place Foley catheters.

Continuous Bladder Irrigation

If the Foley is placed for the reason of too much blood or blood clots in your urine, you will need *continuous bladder irrigation*. Irrigation is achieved through a specialized Foley catheter with three lumens (channels) so that the Foley can be held in place, fluid can be put up into your bladder, and fluid can be drained out to clear the blood. It is placed the same way as a regular Foley.

Post-Void Residual Sonography

If the health care team is worried that after you urinate your bladder has not emptied completely, they will do an ultrasound over the bladder. The *post-void residual sonography* is a very simple, noninvasive procedure in which the ultrasound technician puts a small amount of ultrasound jelly on the skin of your lower abdomen and moves a small probe across your skin over the bladder. Through this procedure the doctor can estimate the amount of urine still in your bladder.

SO Many Kinds of Tests

We have attempted to explain the most common tests encountered during an inpatient stay. Other tests are most often performed in the outpatient setting. This is not a complete and exhaustive list. The good news is that as the field of medicine advances and technology improves, more and more ways to diagnose illnesses are coming to the fore. If you or your family member undergoes a test not explained in these pages, do not hesitate to ask your doctor or nurse to explain the test and also to refer you to more information about the test so that you will be educated. Here is a list of tests not usually performed during an inpatient stay. Occasionally, however, these tests may be done while the patient is in the hospital: kidney biopsy, nerve and muscle conduction testing, positron emission tomography (PET) scan, PFTs (pulmonary function tests).

Cystoscopy

If a look inside your bladder is required, you will have a test called a *cystoscopy*. Usually you do not need to be sedated for this test; in fact, most urologists do this procedure multiple times a day in their offices. You are often given some numbing medication at the area, and a thin scope is inserted up your urethra and into your bladder. The scope is attached to a camera screen so that the doctor can visualize the inside of the bladder, take some pictures, and obtain samples of tissue for analysis.

Lithotripsy

If you have a kidney or ureteral stone that is obstructing the flow of urine, you may require a *lithotripsy.* This is a procedure in which shock waves are directed at the stones to break them up finely so that they can be passed in the urine. The procedure can be done in two ways. In one method you are positioned in a warm water bath, and in the other you sit on top of a soft surface. You are usually given some kind of anesthesia so you are more comfortable and can sit still to tolerate the procedure, which can take about an hour.

Vascular Surgery

Ankle-Brachia Index (ABI) Analysis

Some people suffer from *peripheral arterial disease (PAD),* a narrowing of the arteries. The symptoms of this disease can be manifested by pain in your legs when walking. The *ankle-brachia index (ABI)* is a test that compares the blood pressure in your ankle to the blood pressure in your arm. When the pressure reading is lower in your arms than in your ankles, PAD will be suspected.

Doppler

If there is concern about the blood flow to a part of your body—particularly your legs or feet—you may need to undergo a *Doppler.* This test is an ultrasound that shows the blood flow in your limbs. Often the results of this test are combined with the results of an ABI to help determine the next course of action. A Doppler can also help to determine if you have a blood clot in one of your limbs—otherwise known as a *DVT,* or *deep vein thrombosis.* If the doctor is looking for blood flow of the large arteries in your neck that supply blood to the brain (the *carotids*), you might get a carotid Doppler. Knowing the degree of *stenosis* (blockage) in your carotid arteries can help the doctor and others caring for you determine the risk of stroke.

CHAPTER 9

Nutrition in the Hospital

Many patients are on special diets. Generally, the hospital dietary depart-ment is very thorough and organized about providing the appropriate meals. However, you can help to ensure that you are receiving the trays best suited to your specific nutritional needs. Please think about what spe-cial restrictions you may have. Is sodium (salt) restricted? Are you watch-ing fats and cholesterol for a heart condition? If you are scheduled for a procedure, are you supposed to be eating at all? Older patients may be reluctant to challenge the meals brought to them. Many older folks were raised in an era when you ate what was put in front of you; to do otherwise was considered poor manners. When your health is involved, it isn't rude to question or refuse the wrong tray.

TIP What If the Food on Your Tray Doesn't Look Quite Right?

It sometimes takes a day or so for the correct dietary instructions and re-strictions to be communicated to the dietary department. Unfortunately, this delay has the potential to be harmful to you if your medical condition can be worsened by the wrong food. For example, if you are diabetic and you notice high-sugar content meals being delivered, please say some-thing. You may let your nurse know or speak directly to the individual who delivers the trays.

If you notice you are not being fed at all, ask why. If you notice you are sent only a liquid (or clear) diet—for example, gelatin, ginger ale, clear broth—ask when the diet is to be *advanced* (changed to a more challenging level, in this case a more regular consistency). It will be important to know the reason behind the restriction and whether it is at the request of your health care provider or simply an oversight by the dietary department.

NPO

NPO stands for a Latin phrase, *non per os,* meaning nothing by mouth. You might see a sign on a patient's door or wall with these letters. This precaution is taken to warn everyone coming into the room that the patient may not have ANYTHING to eat or drink. The sign serves as a reminder that the patient should not be fed even if the orders are clearly written in a chart. There might be several reasons for a patient be designated NPO. Commonly, it is because the patient is scheduled for a surgery or a procedure and it would be dangerous to have any food or drink in the stomach. Another reason for NPO orders might be the patient's inability to safely swallow food and drink without risk of choking. The patient may have had a stroke or some other neurological event. Some patients who have pneumonia are suspected of having *aspirated* (inhaled) some food or drink as the cause of the pneumonia. These patients are *contraindicated for* (not allowed) food and drink by mouth. Patients with dementia will have difficulty understanding that they may not even have so much as a sip of water. It will be important to watch over these patients carefully since they are unlikely to integrate this information and consequently to remember that any intake of food or liquid puts them in danger.

Before Procedures and Surgery

Depending on the type of procedure or surgery you are scheduled for, there will be a period of time during which no food or drink is allowed. In other words, you will be NPO. This restriction is done to protect your airway during the surgery or procedure for your own safety. It is extremely important that you comply if food or drink is not permitted. A slight exception to the NPO rule prior to surgery may be made to allow a patient to have a sip of water to take medications. It is important to check with the nurses and doctors to find out if you should take your medications before surgery or other procedures.

Diet after Surgery or a Procedure

Shortly after surgery it is unlikely that you will be allowed to eat. This is because you are waking up from anesthesia, and it is a safety precaution to ensure that you are sufficiently awake and alert to manage eating and drinking. The change of diet after surgery is a very individualized one based on what kind of surgery you have undergone, what organs and body parts were affected, and what diet you were on prior to the surgery or procedure. Typically, food and liquids will be gradually reintroduced. If there has been a very major operation, particularly if any of the digestive organs have been operated on, the reintroduction may be very gradual. During this time, the doctors and nurses will evaluate your readiness for the next step to make sure your digestive tract is prepared for more of a challenge. You might start with clear liquids and ices and then move to pureed solid foods. It could be several days until you are ready for a normal diet. Often after surgery involving the bowels, the doctors and nurses will check you daily to see whether you are making bowel sounds and passing gas. These signs indicate that the bowel is functioning again and ready for the reintroduction of food.

SPEECH AND SWALLOW EVALUATION FOR FEEDING AND DYSPHAGIA DIET

If you have had a stroke or seem to have trouble with speaking and pronunciation—a sign that your tongue muscle is not strong enough to safely direct food down the *esophagus* (food tube) after chewing—you will require a speech and swallow evaluation. This evaluation will usually be performed by a trained speech pathologist.

Dysphagia (difficulty swallowing) is usually determined by a speech and swallow evaluation. Some swallowing difficulties are less severe than others and can be managed with diet modification. A dysphagia diet may also be appropriate if you have difficulty chewing. A dysphagia diet means the food must be of a certain texture, often pureed in a blender, to make it easier to chew and swallow. For patients with dysphagia, the food consistency must be moist and not dry. Liquids can be particularly difficult for some patients to manage safely, since it is possible to aspirate thin liquids—the food goes down the trachea (windpipe) instead of the esophagus (food tube). A thickening agent can be added to any liquid to decrease the risk of aspiration. Dysphagia diets can be confusing, as there are different levels. The speech and swallow therapist will determine the level of diet necessary and will give the nurse specific instructions on how to administer the foods and liquids appropriately. The dietitian or nutritionist is invaluable in ensuring that when you are on a specialized diet you consume enough calories. This health care professional is also an excellent resource for answering any questions you may have about this specialized diet. If you are on the dysphagia diet, you may be discharged to home or a skilled nursing facility with instructions for continued vigilance. You may need to have a conversation with the dietitian (or nutritionist) and the speech therapist about how this will occur and what steps need to be taken to ensure continued safe swallowing.

FLUID RESTRICTION

Your health care provider may have a reason to restrict the amount of fluids you should drink. There may be two principal reasons for this. Fluid restriction may be necessary because your *sodium* (salt) level is abnormal or because of swelling. Many conditions can cause your sodium level to be out of balance and consequently may require the monitoring of your fluid intake; examples are heart failure and liver failure. Swelling may be related to one of these conditions or caused by something else and is typically observed in the lower extremities (legs and ankles). Usually when your fluid is restricted, you will be on a *free water* fluid restriction. Free water includes drinks without particles, such as water, carbonated drinks, coffee, and tea. Milk is an example of a fluid that is not considered free water since it contains solids.

CARDIAC DIET

Patients with heart conditions may be prescribed a cardiac diet. The best way to fight cardiovascular disease is by losing weight, lowering blood pressure, and controlling cholesterol. Cardiac diets are usually low in fat and cholesterol and may be sodium (salt) restricted. If this is a new diet for you, you will need to speak with the dietitian. A dietitian can help you understand which aspects of the diet are most important and what specific foods to avoid or eat sparingly. If you have congestive heart failure, it will be important to adhere to a low-salt diet to prevent fluid retention.

LOW-FIBER DIET

Another term for fiber is *residue*. Fiber is difficult for the colon to break down into digestible components and is important for a properly functioning digestive system. When the colon is inflamed in conditions such as *gastroenteritis*, *diverticulitis*, and *inflammatory bowel disease*, it is unable to break down fiber successfully. During flare-ups or severe intestinal problems, a low-fiber diet puts less stress on the colon. Foods allowed on a low-fiber diet include white bread, rice, white pasta, tender meats, poultry and fish, well-cooked vegetables and fruits without skin or seeds. Foods NOT allowed include whole grains, tough meats, raw vegetables, nuts, seeds, beans, and popcorn. Dairy foods may be eaten as tolerated.

Low Fiber, High Fiber

This was the second time Tom had been hospitalized for diverticulitis. He had been so careful with his doctor's instructions the first time around. Particularly after his colonoscopy and follow-up visit, he had increased the amount of fiber in his diet. He now understood that diverticulitis was the result of a lifelong diet low in fiber. So now that he was feeling better after a few days in the hospital, he wondered why he was put on a low-fiber diet. Tom added this question to his list to ask the doctor and nurse. And sure enough, there was an answer: he learned that a low-fiber diet was necessary while his bowel was still inflamed so that it would heal more easily. When the inflammation calmed down and his condition was resolved, he could go back to his regular high-fiber diet.

DIABETES DIET

Depending on the type of diabetes (type 1 or type 2), individuals with diabetes either do not make *insulin* or are resistant to insulin. Insulin helps the body to process *glucose* (sugar). People with diabetes need a specific diet called a consistent carbohydrate diet (carbohydrates are sugars as well). In a consistent carbohydrate diet each meal has a specified number of grams of carbohydrates. Understanding how many carbohydrates are in each meal and knowing the premeal *blood glucose* level allows you and your health care providers to adjust the dose of insulin properly. If the diabetic diet is something new since hospital admission, you will need detailed instructions from the dietitian or nutritionist.

VITAMIN K AND ANTICOAGULANTS

There are many medical conditions that require the blood to be thinned so that it does not easily clot. *Atrial fibrillation,* a heart arrhythmia, is a common example. Patients with this condition are at increased risk of stroke. Patients with certain types of heart valves, some types of recent operations, and previous blood clots are also required to remain on *anticoagulant* (blood thinning) medication for varying durations, depending on the condition. Blood clotting is a complicated process that involves many different factors found in the blood. Certain factors are dependent on vitamin K to function properly to help blood clotting occur. Vitamin K is a fat-soluble vitamin found in many foods, particularly leafy green vegetables. A blood thinner that is often given to thin the blood is warfarin (known by the brand name Coumadin). Warfarin is a *vitamin K antagonist;* it prevents the proper functioning of certain clotting factors and acts to thin the blood. Patients taking a vitamin K antagonist blood thinner such as warfarin must be careful about their consumption of foods rich in vitamin K as they will counteract the effects of the medication. There are many new anticoagulant medications now approved and available that do not require monitoring vitamin K food intake. You may want to ask your health care providers about what your anticoagulant medication options are.

TIP   Diet for Patients on Warfarin (Coumadin)

Warfarin is a vitamin K antagonist. In order for this drug to be effective, patients must monitor their intake of foods high in vitamin K. Many people think this means they must avoid leafy green vegetables altogether. Often patients can be heard saying they can't eat any more salad, but this is not the case. Instead, it is important to be consistent about the daily intake of vitamin K rich foods. If you have been prescribed warfarin during the hospital stay, you may need to discuss your diet with the nurse, nutritionist, or dietitian.

ALTERNATE FEEDING ROUTES

NG (Nasogastric) Tube Feeding

If you are awake and have the ability to swallow, you will be fed a pre-scribed diet according to your nutritional needs, restrictions, and condition. If you are awake but unable to swallow or if you are sedated and on a breathing machine, feeding may occur through a *nasogastric tube* (*NG tube*). An NG tube is a thin flexible tube that is placed through your nostril and threaded down your esophagus (food tube) and resides in your stomach. The NG tube allows you to be fed with a liquid diet until your condition allows a regular diet to be resumed.

TIP   NG Tube Placement and Removal

Placement (insertion) of the NG tube is uncomfortable, but most likely you will adjust to it after a short period. You may also find the removal of the tube uncomfortable. Our advice is to ask the doctor to pull it out fairly quickly.

PEG Feeding

A *PEG* tube is a *percutaneous endoscopic gastrostomy* tube (see chapter 7) that is placed into your stomach through the skin of the abdomen if you have problems with dysphagia (difficulty swallowing) and/or with maintaining an adequate level of nutrition. A PEG tube is placed by a gastroenterologist, a surgeon, or an interventional radiologist. Patients with a PEG tube receive liquid nutrition, known as PEG feeding. This feeding is of two types—continuous or *bolused*. For continuous feeds, the PEG tube is attached to a pump that is similar in appearance to an IV pump. If you are receiving *bolus* feeds, every few hours a certain amount of the nutritional liquid substance will be injected into the PEG tube through a large plastic syringe. The formulation of the liquid food is determined by the dietitian on the basis of your specific medical problems. For example, patients with diabetes receive different formulas than those with kidney disease.

J-Tube Feeds

Some patients need to be fed directly into the small intestine, bypassing the stomach completely. This occurs when there are blockages such as hernias or in patients with pancreatitis (any food put into the stomach has the potential to irritate the pancreas). In these cases, you will have a *jejunostomy tube (J-tube)* placed instead of a PEG tube. Like a PEG tube, a J-tube tube is placed through the skin of the abdomen, but instead of being inserted into your stomach, it is placed into your jejunum (part of the small bowel). The feeding formula will be tailored to your specific conditions and needs. A J-tube is placed by a gastroenterologist, a surgeon, or an interventional radiologist.

Parenteral Nutrition (PN) and Total Parenteral Nutrition (TPN)

Parenteral nutrition (PN) is a form of nutrition that is outside the digestive tract. This route of administration involves piercing the skin or mucous membrane to provide nutrition through the veins by an IV. In contrast to PEG or J-tube feeding (see above), where the food is directly deposited into the stomach or intestines, PN bypasses the gastrointestinal organs. PN is the term used when other forms of feeding are also being utilized. When a patient is receiving no other form of nutrition, it called *total parenteral nutrition (TPN)*. TPN comes with many complications such as infections, blood clots, and fatty liver. For this reason, it is used very sparingly and only when absolutely necessary. Patients will need TPN when they have a nonfunctioning gastrointestinal tract or require complete bowel rest, which may be the case in a bowel obstruction.

DIET IN THE ICU

Your diet in the ICU is determined the same way as your diet on a regular floor (unit). If you are awake and have the ability to swallow, you will be fed a prescribed diet according to your nutritional needs, restrictions, and condition. If you are awake but unable to swallow or if you are sedated and on a breathing machine, feeding will occur through an NG tube. If you are sedated, you will not be bothered by the tube. NG placement is performed by any trained health care professional.

> **TIP**   Dietary Changes May Be Stressful
>
> Patients and families both get stressed when feeding is restricted or a diet is dramatically changed. Be sure to ask questions about the choice of a specific diet and what the plan is for resuming normal feeding. Remember that getting back to a normal diet may take some time. It may be helpful to write down the expected time for the transition. Your nurse will be a good source of information about dietary matters. You might also ask to speak to the dietitian or nutritionist.

NUTRITIONAL SUPPLEMENTS

The body cannot heal without proper nutrition. Some patients are unable or unwilling to take in adequate nutrition and may require nutritional supplements. Nutritional supplementation is a controversial topic since some health care professionals believe in supplements wholeheartedly and think every patient should have them as part of a complete diet, while others believe that they are not well utilized by the body. In the hospital, the most common situation for the addition of nutritional supplements is wound care, since inadequate nutrition may impede healing in these patients. Nutritional supplements are not uniformly accepted as therapeutic; therefore, if they are prescribed, you should have a discussion with your health care team to arrive at a mutual decision.

BRINGING IN FOOD FOR THE PATIENT

We have discussed many different diets for hospitalized patients and the importance of appropriate nutrition. The right diet will help patients recover, while the wrong foods will hinder this process. **For this reason you should not bring in any food for patients unless you have permission from the medical or surgical team.** All too often the doctors and nurses are perplexed about why a patient's blood sugar is high or why the patient is retaining so much fluid only to find out that the family is bringing in food that is not consistent with the prescribed diet. In contrast, there are scenarios in which a family will be encouraged to bring in food if the patient does not enjoy the hospital meals and will eat only a small amount. This can often be the case when the patient is used to eating certain ethnic foods that are not offered in the hospital. In this situation, the health care team may ask the family to bring in food. Naturally, any food items brought in for the patient must be consistent with the type of diet that has been prescribed to suit the patient's specific conditions and needs.

FEEDING THE FAMILY

There will be times when friends and families will "camp out" in the patient's room or the visitor lounges. If there is a very sick patient or if visiting hours are allowed for short periods, visitors may find that they are staying at the hospital for long stretches. Parents of *neonates* (newborns), young children, and adolescents tend to move in with the patient; this is a good thing and will be discussed more fully in the section on the hospitalized child in chapter 12. Regardless of the stress level experienced by having a loved one in the hospital, good nutrition is essential to fuel the body, bolster spirits, and prevent added stress on the body's *homeostatic* (balancing) systems. Visitors are advised to find out the opening hours of the hospital cafeterias and snack shops and to be prepared to bring their own food during the patient's stay. Some floors will make microwave ovens available for visitors; usually there are also microwave ovens in the cafeteria. We stress that it is not always appropriate to share the meals and snacks from home with the patient as there are a multitude of reasons that certain food items are not suited to the patient's nutritional needs and might even be harmful.

TIP Off-Hours Arrival

Hospital dietary service runs on a schedule to feed patients at least three times a day. You will see the cart with covered trays at regular intervals morning, noon, and evening at roughly the same time each day. What if you arrive at your bed at an off-hour, having spent a long time in a holding area in the emergency room, and you are hungry? You may have missed the regular meal delivery, so you must ask the nurse to order a tray or to have some type of nourishment sent up. Some floors will have puddings or other snacks available for exactly this purpose. This might also be the time to alert the nurse about your specific dietary needs and restrictions.

CHAPTER 10

Protocols and Precautions

HOSPITAL RULES

There seem to be many rules in the hospital, and it is likely that not all of them will make sense to you. Be assured that these rules are in place to protect you as well as your privacy and to allow the staff to perform their jobs and functions in the best possible way. Therefore, if visiting hours are short, or there is a limit to how many guests may visit you in the room, this rule is not intended to punish your families and friends but rather to allow you to rest and to create the best conditions that allow the staff to better care for you.

Different types of hospital wards (also called floors or units) have different rules. In the *obstetrical* (maternity) ward, it is common and usually desirable to see a multitude of family friends and even young children. This is because, for the most part, mom and most newborns are healthy and young and not at too much risk for being disturbed or getting ill. The vulnerable patients—the newborn babies with low birth weight or other conditions who may be at risk for getting ill—are, for their protection, in the nursery during visiting times. There, everyone can take delight in seeing them through the safety of a large glass window.

At the extreme other end of the spectrum, patients in the bone marrow transplant unit (or burn unit) must be protected from every possible contaminant and germs. Visitors—when they are allowed—and staff alike will be asked to don masks, gloves, and paper gowns so that they do not carry in anything harmful on clothing or skin. These patients are vulnerable in every way, and you will notice a hush on these floors and signs that no plants are allowed. We discuss this topic in greater detail in chapter 12, on special patient populations.

HAND WASHING

Hand washing is an absolute must for all health care providers. In fact, it is so important that every year all employees in hospitals are tested on their ability to wash their hands properly. They are asked to wash their hands with a special soap; afterward, hands are screened for residual soap. It is best if providers and staff wash their hands in front of you, but this is not always feasible; you may see hospital personnel using hand sanitizer. Many providers will also put gloves on after washing their hands. This is not always necessary, depending on the nature of the interaction with you. However, if a provider physically touches you, he or she should wash their hands before and after. If you haven't seen the health care providers wash their hands, you should feel empowered to ask them whether they have done so, particularly if they have no gloves on. This is crit-

Protocols

What is a *protocol*? It is a set of rules or guidelines designed to help physicians, nurses, and professional staff take care of patients in a standardized, uniform way. In recent years, there has been a great emphasis on helping health care providers perform patient care with as little variation as possible. Once we have learned that something works and is successful, it makes sense to always do it this way. Many of the phenomena encountered in the hospital occur with great frequency. For example, many patients are at risk for falling. To deal with this threat, specific prevention strategies are put in place: warning notes in the medical record (patient chart—be it paper or electronic), signs on the door, bars raised on the bed, and increased alertness by floor staff. Another common but very simple protocol is hand washing. Protocols may be simple or complex. They may be one step or consist of many different activities to ensure patient safety.

ical and it's why many hospitals plaster signs around units suggesting that patients "ask me if I have cleaned my hands."

TIP   Hand Washing

Do not be afraid to ask if the person taking care of you, touching you or
your medical equipment, has cleaned his or her hands. You might say
something like, "I've noticed all sorts of signs suggesting I ask people if
they have washed or cleaned their hands. I'm sure you have and I didn't
notice, but I would just like to make sure."

GI PROPHYLAXIS

GI prophylaxis is also known as *stress ulcer prophylaxis*; it is a preventive
strategy in which you are given stomach acid-lowering medications to reduce the risk of stress ulcers and gastrointestinal (GI) bleeding. Unfortunately, this practice is extremely overutilized in situations where there
is not a clear reason for its use. GI prophylaxis is appropriate for those
patients with the highest risk of GI bleeding, including patients on mechanical ventilation (*intubated*) or who have a *coagulopathy* (a bleeding
disorder).

TIP   GI Prophylaxis Only When Necessary

If you have been prescribed GI prophylaxis such as Prilosec or Protonix
(omeprazole or pantoprazole), ask your doctors and nurses if you are at
high enough risk to warrant its use. These drugs are useful and necessary
for certain patients but not for all. Further, like all drugs, they have the
potential to interact with other medications.

ASPIRATION PREVENTION

You may come into the hospital with swallowing problems or may develop
the problem during the hospital stay as a result of procedures or changes

in your condition. *Aspiration* occurs when food or liquid material taken in by your mouth ends up going down the trachea (windpipe) instead of the esophagus (food pipe). When this happens, there is the potential to develop pneumonia. If you are at risk of aspiration, aspiration precautions will be put in place. One of these measures is to elevate the head section of your bed by at least forty-five degrees. You should be placed upright between forty-five and ninety degrees, particularly while eating and drinking. For health care professionals, there is nothing more frightening than finding a family member feeding an elderly patient who is in a mostly reclined position. Even the best of swallowers could choke in this position. If you are at risk for aspiration, you will likely be evaluated by a speech pathologist to determine what consistency of food and liquids is safe or if you cannot take in food by mouth. We discuss this more fully in the section on speech and swallow evaluation in chapter 9.

DVT OR VTE PROPHYLAXIS

If you've been admitted to the hospital, either for a medical problem or for surgery, you are almost always at a higher risk for developing a blood clot (*venous thromboembolism) (VTE*). A clot results when the blood is not flowing well. Often clots form in the legs, where you may or may not experience symptoms (pain, swelling, redness, tenderness). This is called a *deep vein thrombosis*, or *DVT*. The real danger exists when a clot travels from your legs or arms to one of your lungs. This becomes a life-threatening situation. Certain factors and conditions, such as older age, immobility, prior clots, obesity, heart failure, respiratory illness, inflammatory bowel disease, and current active cancer put you at higher risk for developing a clot. In addition, hip and knee replacement surgery and abdominal cancer surgery raise this risk. For many reasons, being in a hospital increases the risk as well. Recently there has been a great deal of interest in preventing blood clots because they are seen as a large patient safety issue. Most hospitals have a protocol in place to evaluate your risk for clots and to give you medications or to put specialized appliances on you. If the doctor or nurses determine that you are among patients at highest risk for developing a clot (and most hospitalized people are), if there are no reasons that interfere, you will be prescribed VTE or DVT *prophylaxis* injections or pills of anti-coagulant (blood-thinning) medication. Examples of these medications include warfarin (brand name Coumadin), heparin, enoxaparin (brand name Lovenox), fondaparinux (brand name Arixtra), and rivaroxaban (brand name Xarelto). Of course, if you are already on a blood thinner for ANY reason at home or in a skilled nursing facility, then you are already protected against clots. For some patients, the risk of bleeding outweighs the risk of clots. Examples are injury to the head, certain types of surgery, gastrointestinal bleeding, very low platelet count, and anemia due to bleeding. For these patients mechanical prophylaxis will be ordered. Machines known as *sequential compression devices* (*SCD*, brand name Venodynes) surround your legs and periodically compress them to keep the blood flowing well; they are used while you are in bed. There are also *compression stockings* (*TEDS*, or thromboembolism-deterrent hose) that can be worn when you are not in bed. If clinically indicated and safe for you, vigorous and constant walking will also help to reduce the risk of clots.

PREVENTION OF FALLS

Falls may be a serious complication during the hospital stay and can be life-threatening. For a variety of reasons, you are often at risk for falling during your stay in the hospital. For patients at risk prior to admission, this risk will probably be exacerbated by a hospital stay. Many medications cause dizziness and drowsiness. You may be on new medications, administered to you in the hospital, and you may be feeling new effects at the start. You may be on sleeping or pain medications, including narcotics, which cause lightheadedness and dizziness. You may be disoriented and confused. You may be deconditioned by weakness since the longer you stay in bed, the more difficult it is for you to swing back into normal activities. Muscles not used to moving, particularly in older patients, do not support the body well. A fall has the potential to cause broken bones, serious bruising, and more illness. It can have devastating consequences if you are receiving anticoagulation medication for treatment or prevention since you will be at higher risk for bleeds. For all these reasons, extra care must be taken when you move out of the bed. If you are at extremely high risk of falling, there may be a sign on your door or over your bed alerting everyone that you are a fall risk. This reminds anyone who comes into the room to reinstate or raise the bars on the side of the bed in the upright position.

> **TIP**   For Patients at Risk of Falling
>
> Patients who are at risk for falling must never try to leave the bed without help. Friends and family might need to be very firm about this. If you believe that your family member is dizzy, weak, or in some way unsteady on his or her feet, tell the nurse, the nurse's aides (patient care associates), and the doctors about your concern. Remember that you may be the most alert about your loved one—you are the first line of defense. If your family member is designated as a fall risk, you may want to consider spending extra time at the hospital and enlisting friends and family to keep watch. On a busy patient floor, with staff pulled in many directions caring for multiple sick patients, it is impossible to have eyes and ears on everyone. You may need to help reinforce the warning that your family member needs assistance when getting out of bed.

ISOLATION

You will be put into isolation either to protect yourself against infection or to prevent others from being exposed to your highly contagious illness.

Reverse Isolation

If you have cancer, HIV AIDS, a bone marrow transplant, or a weakened immune system, you must be protected from infection. Your body has an inability to fend off infection; this condition is referred to as *immunocompromised*. Visitors to immunocompromised patients may be asked to wear a mask and possibly a gown. This is considered *reverse isolation*.

Negative Pressure Isolation

If you have a highly contagious respiratory illness such as tuberculosis (TB) or chicken pox, your illness may be spread through the air. To decrease the spread of these illnesses, you may be placed in *negative pressure isolation,* in a *negative pressure room*, which allows the air to enter, but not to exit, the room. Anyone—staff and visitors alike—entering your room will have to put on a special fitted mask.

Flu, *C. diff.,* and MRSA

Following are descriptions of three *pathogens* (germs) that are common to hospitals and require special prevention measures.

Influenza (Flu)
During the fall and winter months in particular, hospitals must take special precautions to guard against *influenza* (flu) because of its ability to spread rapidly and its life-threatening potential for certain patient groups (the very young, the elderly, and the immunocompromised). The flu is a highly contagious virus that is usually spread through the air by coughing or sneezing. It may also be transmitted by touching a surface contaminated with the virus. During active flu season, it is also important that health care providers wash their hands before and after seeing each patient, to kill influenza that gets on the skin. To prevent contracting airborne flu, health care providers will wear masks to protect themselves when seeing a patient who has or is presumed to have the flu. Most hospitals have protocols in place for all personnel to be vaccinated against the flu and to display this vaccination status on their ID badges. It is now required in some hospitals for providers and staff who did not get the flu shot to wear a mask at all times while in patient areas. During flu season, patients who did not receive a flu vaccine prior to admission may be offered a vaccine at the time of discharge.

C. diff. and Contact Precautions
C. diff. (Clostridium difficile) are bacteria normally found in the gut and usually do not cause problems. However, antibiotics, while killing the bad bacteria that sicken, also kill many of the normal *flora* (bacteria) in the colon. When the normal flora are killed, *C.diff.* bacteria have a tendency to take over and multiply. This leads to a bad case of diarrhea, which is characterized by multiple watery, foul-smelling episodes. *C. diff.* diarrhea is contagious, transmitted through feces, and can spread very quickly from patient to patient if health care workers are not diligent about following

the proper precautions. It is important to know that **hand sanitizers do not kill these bacteria**. Good old-fashioned hand washing with soap and hot water will kill the bacteria. If you have *C. diff.*, everyone who enters the room must take these precautions, including wearing disposable gowns and gloves. This type of prevention protocol is called *contact precautions,* and there will be a special sign on the door to alert visitors and staff.

MRSA and Contact Precautions

MRSA stands for *methicillin-resistant Staphylococcus aureus* and is often referred to as the superbug. You may have heard or read about superbugs in the media. In plain language, this means MRSA is a type of bacteria normally found on your skin that has developed resistance to many antibiotics. When bacteria develop resistance, they are harder to treat since the choices of antibiotics are limited. MRSA is spread through contact and can be transmitted easily in the hospital because patients with weakened immune systems are more susceptible to it. A patient with an active MRSA infection may be placed on contact precautions requiring staff and visitors to wear gown and gloves.

PAIN MANAGEMENT SERVICE

There are many different ways to manage your pain in the hospital. There are times when your pain is so severe that it may require the expertise of a pain management service. This service is usually made up of a doctor and nurse or nurse practitioner with additional training in pain management. They are equipped with the knowledge to prescribe, monitor, and adjust high-dose pain medications; use alternative methods such as epidural steroid injections; and regulate PCA (patient-controlled analgesic) pumps. PCA pumps are often used if you've just had surgery or if you are in intolerable pain from other conditions such as sickle cell crisis.

LIFT EQUIPMENT

Nurses, patient care associates (nurse's aides), and hospital *orderlies* put their own physical health at risk every day on the job in the hospital. This is because they are often responsible for rolling and transferring patients. Their most common injuries are musculoskeletal, with back injury in the lead. Many hospitals have protocols in place to try to protect nurses and other employees who are moving patients. Special equipment such as a mechanical lift needs to be used when patients can't move at all themselves and to help lift patients who cannot support their own weight. Even patients who are not obese may pose a risk of injury to hospital personnel. Do not be offended if you are moved with the help of a mechanical assistive lift device.

RESTRAINTS

The use of restraints in the hospital is a topic of heated debate. Sometimes patients can become so agitated that they put themselves at risk for harm. When someone is delusional, confused, or in pain, he or she may exhibit impulsive behaviors such as ripping out IV lines or pulling out Foley catheters and nasogastric tubes. Restraints are generally used as a last resort to keep the patient safe; most hospitals have a strict restraint policy. First and foremost, every attempt is made to reorient patients and make environmental adjustments to decrease their confusion. When a patient is unable to be calmed down, the choices of restraints can be physical or chemical. Under specific circumstances, a vest or only soft two-point restraints placed around the wrist—as opposed to hard four-point restraints, on all four limbs—can be used. An up-to-date hospital will have a strict policy about how long the restraints can be on before the patient is reassessed by a nurse or doctor; this prevents patients from being restrained for days. A chemical restraint is a sedating medication that can be ordered only by a doctor or other qualified medical professional; common ones are lorazepam (Ativan) and haloperidol (Haldol). However, the use of these medications should be very limited in elderly patients, and therefore medication is not always the best solution.

PREVENTING DELIRIUM

The best way to prevent delirium is to anticipate it in advance and then use the best methods possible to head it off. Most patients with any level—including a low level—of dementia are at a high risk for delirium. Patients receiving pain medication or sedatives are at risk as well. To prevent delirium, the key is to control the patient's environment to optimize orientation. Day versus night cues are extremely important; therefore, patients separated from a window by a curtain are not getting these cues. At-risk patients will also need to have as many of their "faculties" as possible to keep them oriented; glasses, dentures, and hearing aids will help prevent delirium.

Here are some steps family members can take to help prevent delirium in an at-risk patient:

- Advocate for your family member to be moved to a bed by the window.
- Be sure to frequently reorient your loved one with all their assistive devices.
- Consider asking for a geriatric consultation if you find your family member confused and sometimes restrained.

Restraints

In past decades, agitated patients would be tied to the bed with hard leather restraints at four points: both wrists and both lower legs. This medieval-sounding practice might have made things easier for the nurses, but it was uncomfortable and even cruel for the patient and in certain instances caused some fatalities. Fortunately, restraint "punishment" at four points or with a straitjacket is no longer deemed acceptable. In the current era, patient-centered care is valued over staff convenience.

TIP   Patients with Dementia

If your family member has dementia, even if only the beginning stages, it is important to let the doctors and nurses know. If you have noticed periods of confusion at home with your family member, tell the doctor or nurse caring for him or her. Has your family member been hospitalized before and had episodes of delirium? It is important to share this information. The health care team will be most successful at working with you if they understand the patient's *baseline* (how he or she was before admission).

Put Yourself in the Patient's Shoes

Imagine that you have become ill or have a sudden need for surgery; you are not feeling at your best. Imagine that you had some confusion already and then you were placed in a two-bed or four-bed room and your bed was near the door. By the door, you have no access to the window, so you lose track of whether it is day or night. By the door, it is loud because of the proximity to the hallway and its activity. Now you are having trouble sleeping at night because of hall noise. During the day, you catch up on your sleep and pretty soon, you have your days and nights mixed up. Soon you can become delirious—we used to refer to this confusion in the evening as *sundowning*. Imagine also that you are without your glasses, hearing aids, or dentures. It is difficult enough to be in the hospital, to be sick, or to be recovering from surgery. Now you really cannot fathom what is going on around you.

PRESSURE ULCERS (BEDSORES)

Humans weren't meant to lie in one spot all day. Through receptors in the skin, the body senses when you have been on one spot for too long, and you are prompted to change positions. Immobilized patients lying in one spot for prolonged periods will ultimately develop *pressure ulcers* (bedsores). Pressure ulcers are difficult to heal; therefore, there is a great effort to prevent them from forming. When you are admitted to the hospital, you will have your skin evaluated for preexisting pressure ulcers, which are classified as stage 1 through stage 4. Stage 1 is a non-*blanching* (whitening after pressure) redness of the skin. Stage 2 is an open ulcer only partway through the top part of skin. Stage 3 is loss of all the tissue of the skin right above the layer of fat and bone. Stage 4 describes a sore in which you can see muscle or bone. The only way to effectively prevent pressure ulcers is with frequent (every two hours) turning. There are also skin protectors that can be placed over vulnerable spots such as the heels. Nurses are very experienced with pressure ulcer prevention and treatment; they will document evidence of any pressure ulcers and will note the stage. If your family member has a pressure ulcer that is not healing, you can request a consultation with a wound-care expert. Whole books by nursing researchers and scholars have been written on the medical management of pressure ulcers. We encourage you to explore these additional resources if you have a family member who has, or is at risk of having, pressure ulcers.

BED REST VERSUS MOBILIZATION

People are in the hospital for a variety of medical or surgical reasons. In certain cases they will have instructions to remain in bed—this is called bed rest. Decades ago most hospitalized patients were placed on bed rest for a prolonged period of time. It was felt that this allowed the body to heal. We now know that prolonged bed rest when unnecessary can actually cause harm to a patient. Patients can develop blood clots, pneumonia, bedsores, and a slowing down of the digestive system. Bed rest may be appropriate in specific situations, at specific times, and for specific patients. For example, after certain surgical procedures, walking may be dangerous and may compromise recovery. The doctors and nurses will determine what level of mobilization is safe and appropriate for your case, taking into account many different factors. If you are unsure about your bed rest status, please ask the health care team.

Early Mobilization

Most patients will be surprised how quickly they will be asked to get out of bed and start *ambulating* (walking). For most patients, the earlier they get out of bed, the sooner they will be on the road to recovery. More and more, hospitals are recognizing that not just walking but aggressive early walking soon after admission can benefit you and speed your recovery. Many patients will need some kind of assistance with getting out of bed and moving, especially at first. Nurses, patient care associates, family members, and physical therapists may all be called upon to help. You might require a walker or another assistive device. In consultation with nurses and physical therapists, the doctor will advise you and your family members when it is safe to walk unassisted. As always, the benefit of getting up and walking will be weighed against the risk of falls.

Physical Therapy

If you have had orders for bed rest and new orders are written for you to start walking, you may need to be assessed on your ability to do this safely. A physical therapist will get you out of bed and determine how well you can walk and how much assistance you need. Some people won't be able to actually walk for a while, but a physical therapist can still work with that patient to do range-of-motion exercises and help to prevent muscle *atrophy* (wasting or weakening). Muscles not used quickly can become weak and increase the time it takes for you to become independent at walking again. The physical therapist will also determine whether at the time of discharge you need to go to a rehabilitation facility or can return home with or without physical therapy.

Get Up and Get Moving!

Ross was recovering from open-heart surgery. Ouch. The surgeon had sawed through his sternum to bypass the vessels in his heart. He had had tubes inserted in many body places. Everything hurt! He had spent nearly twenty-four hours in an intensive care unit. Now he was going to move to the step-down unit. Time to get out of bed. Time to walk. Ouch. Every day the

Bed Rest—Is It Reasonable in the Year 2017?

Older readers may recall that decades ago, sick people were advised to rest in order to get better. "Sick" also meant recovering from surgery, which is different from how we understand many operations today. The thinking about bed rest has radically changed. Your doctor and nurses very often will want you to get up and walk RIGHT AWAY. Even if you are too weakened to walk, you will have to shuffle two steps to a chair to slowly get used to getting out of bed. We now understand that bed rest may be one of the least helpful ways for hospitalized patients to recover. Patients who linger in bed are at risk for blood clots, pneumonia, constipation, urinary catheters, muscle wasting, and confusion. So if you are asked to get out of bed and walk, put on a smile as you circle the nurses' station and know that the more you move, the sooner you will get better. If you are a family member or patient's friend, encourage the patient to get moving.

nurses and doctors encouraged him to walk a little longer and little farther. How was this possible? Did they wish him harm? Quite the opposite: we know now that reconditioning and moving is the path to recovery from all types of illness and operations.

RAPID RESPONSES

There are situations in the hospital that will require the urgent attention of hospital personnel. Any serious changes in your condition can warrant the staff to call what is known as a rapid response. A rapid response is a protocol that will immediately alert a team of providers, usually doctors and nurses affiliated with either the intensive care unit or hospital medicine. These providers can quickly assess a patient situation and determine what course of action needs to be taken—for example, whether oxygen is needed, whether different medications are indicated, or whether you should be transferred to a higher level of care within the hospital. Most institutions empower all hospital personnel, patients, and visitors to ask for a rapid response to be called if there is a change in the patient's condition. Examples that warrant a rapid response are difficulty breathing, chest pain, and alteration in mental status.

CODES

If a patient is found to have stopped breathing or to be in *cardiac arrest* (heart stopped), a *code* will be called. A code goes by different names in different hospitals. Sometimes it is called a "999" or a "code blue," and it is announced over the intercom. The nearest responder in the hospital will start doing CPR until the code team arrives. Other types of codes can be called for stroke, trauma, pediatric emergencies, and neonatal emergencies. Each code type will alert the medical or surgical team best suited to managing the emergency. It is not always possible for visitors to distinguish the type of code called over the intercom; however, hospital personnel are trained to know the different codes and to respond with great speed.

CHAPTER 11

Intensive Care Units (ICUs)

Intensive care units, commonly called ICUs and also referred to as critical care and special care units, are just that: specialized floors in the hospital for patients who need *monitoring* (extra attention) for some reason. Walking into an ICU can be quite a frightening experience. If you are admitted to one of these units, it means that you are critically ill. There are many different types of ICUs in the hospital depending on the nature of the illness and the type of treatment required. A community hospital may have one combined ICU or no ICU at all. At the other end of the spectrum, a tertiary care or academic medical center will have many different types of ICUs to serve the diverse needs of its patients. If it turns out that your local hospital does not have the appropriate facilities or specialized services to care for you, it is possible that you will be transferred to a hospital with more services. However, this can be done only if you are medically stable for a transfer.

MONITORING

A specific feature of intensive care is enhanced monitoring—particularly by ICU nurses, who will use their training and experience to watch you carefully. You will also be hooked up to many different kinds of machines, and you will likely have many tubes and lines going in and out of your body. Typically in the ICU, your vital functions will be transmitted to the nursing desk or station by computer screens and displayed on monitors by the bedside. Depending on your condition, different functions will be monitored. Generally, blood pressure, temperature, pulse rate, oxygen saturation, and heart rhythm will be displayed, but central venous pressure and pulmonary pressures may be tracked for certain conditions. It is almost impossible for a nonexpert to interpret these readings, so rest assured that if something goes wrong, an alarm bell will sound to bring staff into the room. Sometimes the alarm goes off simply because of a battery failure or a patient's moving a certain way. Although this may be scary for family members, the ICU staff is well trained to respond to the important sounds.

AMBIANCE IN THE ICU

You will likely hear a lot of beeping and buzzing of life-sustaining machines and monitoring devices in the ICU, but you will not hear the kind of chatter observed on other floors (wards, units). There are several reasons for this:

Patients are sedated or asleep to recover from illness or surgery.
There often are no TVs on or patients using their cell phones.
There are fewer visitors (and almost no children) because of limited visiting hours.
Health professionals are focused on taking care of very sick patients.

PHYSICAL LAYOUT OF THE ICU

Most ICUs look different from other units (wards, floors) in the hospital: there is more glass, and nursing pods or stations are closer to the patient rooms. (Current ICU design has individual rooms for all patients.) Patients may appear to be more "on display." This can be disturbing to the observer. However, there is a very good reason for keeping patients within the sight lines of the health professionals. ICU patients typically need constant surveillance and monitoring. Although there will be computer screens to furnish information and alarms to ring if something changes with the set of vital functions, nothing takes the place of the watchful attention of the nurses, doctors, PAs, and NPs. If privacy is required for procedures, washing, toileting, or family conferences, curtains can be pulled temporarily. We will admit that despite an effort to prevent it, patients in the ICU may suffer a certain loss of dignity. This may be more upsetting to friends and family than to the patients themselves. Current efforts are under way to minimize this by allowing greater visitation and by permitting family members to be present throughout the ICU stay, including all procedures. This change is already in place at some hospitals throughout the United States, and the acceptance of this practice appears to be growing.

Perhaps you will notice the absence of patient bathrooms in a typical ICU. Most ICU rooms have a pull-out toilet. However, these toilets are infrequently used since most patients in the ICU are semi-immobile. Toileting is usually done with a bedpan and/or portable urinal, and many patients have a *Foley* (urinary) or rectal catheter inserted at least temporarily.

SPECIAL MEDICATIONS IN THE ICU

There are certain drugs that are typically administered in a monitored setting. One of the most common examples is a class of drugs called *pressors*. Pressors are given to patients who have a blood pressure that is too low to adequately supply blood flow to necessary organs. A blood pressure that is too low is not compatible with life. Common pressors are dobutamine and norepinephrine. Other highly specialized medications used in the ICU include neuromuscular paralytic agents and insulin drips.

NUTRITION IN THE ICU

Nutrition is an essential part of healing and will be addressed for all patients in the ICU. Many ICU patients will not be able to eat normally for safety or logistical reasons. Sedated patients and those on a *ventilator* (breathing machine) or with swallowing issues will receive an *NG* or other *enteric* (relating to the intestines) tube through which liquid food can be administered. In extreme circumstances, some patients are fed through a venous line—this is called *parenteral nutrition (PN)* or *total parenteral nutrition (TPN)*. See chapter 9 for descriptions of different ways that patients may be fed.

VISITING HOURS

Most ICUs will have designated visiting hours. These are usually much more restricted than on the general inpatient wards. Most ICUs have *interdisciplinary rounds* a few times a day, with different specialties and professionals discussing each patient situation. These rounds can take quite a long time as each detail of every patient's care is addressed. While the ICU has fewer patients than the floors, each patient is critically ill and requires a tremendous amount of time and resources. Please plan on finding out when visiting hours are and when will be the best time to speak to the physician and other care team members about any questions you have.

NURSING RATIOS

One of the biggest differences between any ICU and a general unit is the number of nurses working to take care of patients. In an ICU, because patients need more attention, there might be anywhere from one nurse assigned per patient to one nurse taking care of three or four patients at a time. This is in contrast to the number of patients cared for on a generalized non-intensive care unit. Nationally, we have seen estimates of the patient-to-nurse ratio as 2.5 to 3 in most ICUs and the patient-to-nursing-assistant ratio as 4 to 1.However, there will be wide variation across hospitals, types of ICUs, and regions. This staffing arrangement can be a dynamic situation; if a sicker patient is admitted to an ICU, nursing ratios will be rearranged to accommodate patient needs. Conversely, as patients recover and prepare to move to less intensive care, the nursing level of attention may decrease. ICU nurses have extra training to take care of critically ill patients. Their work is difficult and requires constant focus and attention. Further, not all patients recover, and this sense of futility may impose emotional strain on the nurses and assistants involved in their care. For all these reasons, although it may not be evident to the observer, the rates of nursing burnout are higher in ICUs.

TIP   Nursing Ratios in ICUs

Attentive, focused nursing care keeps ICU patients safe. Ideally, the nurse-to-patient ratio should be one to one or one to two for most critically ill patients, depending on the severity of the patient's illness and requirements for care. But this is not always the case. For family members who notice that the ratios are one to three or even one to four, your patient may be in danger. This is the time to advocate on behalf of your loved one; start with the nurse manager to say that you have concerns about the amount of attention the patient is receiving. If this conversation does not bring the desired results, speak with the attending physician or ICU medical director. Finally, if necessary, you may need to approach hospital administration.

ICU PROTOCOLS

Certain aspects of an inpatient stay in an ICU are quite different from those in a stay on a normal medical or surgical floor. Since patients are sicker, less mobile, and more vulnerable, hospitals are attuned to creating specialized measures to protect them. These measures or guidelines are termed *protocols*. We describe them below.

Ventilator and Weaning Protocols

Often in the ICU, patients need the help of a ventilator to breathe. A ventilator is a machine that breathes for you. Taking care of patients on ventilator support requires special training. Usually one of the doctors responsible for overseeing patients on ventilators is trained in pulmonary medicine; the nurses have extra training as well. Respiratory therapists are key personnel on these units since their specialty is precisely geared to caring for ventilated patients. This expertise is important because complications can arise. Patients on ventilators are at very high risk for contracting pneumonia; therefore, preventing this serious illness is a focus. Getting patients off the ventilator so that they do not become dependent on mechanical breathing is a prime objective. This is a complex practice that depends on many

factors to be assessed by the health care team, including proper functioning of the muscles that control breathing, ability to breathe spontaneously,
and discontinuation of certain drugs. The practice of removing patients
from ventilators is called *weaning*; some patients wean easily, while others require more time. There are usually protocols to determine weaning
readiness since putting patients back on the "vent" is associated with poor
outcomes. Patients who require chronic ventilatory support will usually be
moved to a respiratory care unit or to intermediate care units.

Sedation Vacations

Often patients in the ICU need to be sedated (put to sleep artificially) for
their safety and to give their bodies time to heal. Some ICUs have protocols whereby they give the patient a *sedation vacation,* which may also be
a drug holiday. The patient is removed from sedation for a short period
of time; this is often a good opportunity to assess the patient's neurologic
function, including mental status. It is believed that interrupting sedating
drugs may be helpful in preventing ICU *delirium.*

ICU Delirium

Almost two-thirds of patients in the ICU get ICU delirium. Delirium is
an altered state of consciousness that waxes and wanes. That means that
one minute the patient may seem like his or her normal self and the next
minute may act confused. Signs of ICU delirium can be confusion, agitation, decreased attention span, trouble sleeping, and depression. Some
patients are more susceptible to ICU delirium: the elderly, those with
dementia, those on a ventilator, and those with certain medical illnesses
both chronic and acute. Though in the past ICU delirium was not a well
recognized entity, there is currently much attention focused on prevention, and staff in most ICUs are trained to recognize the symptoms; many
ICUs have protocols to prevent or diminish its occurrence.

Infection Control

Enough cannot be said about the need for preventing infection for patients in the ICU. There are entire books written about the process of

infection control in the ICU. Every time a doctor, nurse, NP, or PA performs a procedure, inserts a line, or examines the patient, there is an infection prevention protocol that must be followed. Infections have become such a serious problem that hospitals these days are tracked on the number of hospital-acquired conditions each month. Common infections include *catheter-associated urinary tract infections (CAUTI)* and *central line-associated blood stream infections (CLABSI)*. Some advanced ICUs are equipped with video monitoring to ensure that ICU personnel wash their hands upon entering and leaving patient rooms. Depending on the type of procedure or intervention required and the type of infection a patient has, care providers will need to wear gowns, gloves, face masks, and eye protection equipment. Visitors may also be asked to wear disposable gowns if the patient has a contagious infectious disease. Visitors will be instructed by the nursing staff as to the proper precautions.

SPECIALIZED ICUs

Following are descriptions of types of ICUs that are present in some hospitals.

Medical Intensive Care Unit (MICU)

The *medical intensive care unit (MICU)* is where adult patients with severe general medical issues are taken care of. As with all the ICUs, some patients are admitted to this specialized unit because they need a higher level of observation. Other patients may be there because they are critically ill and require ventilators and special medications to maintain their blood pressure (pressors). This unit is equipped to take care of all critical medical problems and is run by a doctor with advanced training in critical care. This is often an internist who has done a fellowship (extra year or years of training) in pulmonary and/or critical care, but it can also be a nephrologist (kidney doctor), anesthesiologist, emergency room physician, or other specialist.

Surgical Intensive Care Unit (SICU)

The *surgical intensive care unit (SICU)* is very similar to the MICU in terms of layout and nursing care, with the exception that surgeons lead the interdisciplinary team in this unit. The SICU is where patients with surgical complications or possibly very complex, long surgeries are taken care of. Some examples of a surgical complication are infections or heavy bleeding or ruptured internal organs. Surgeons may choose to have their patients admitted to the SICU if a surgery did not go as planned or if the patient was very compromised (ill) before surgery. A perfectly healthy patient with a very long *elective* (planned) surgery (such as scoliosis correction) may need extra attention and therefore may end up in the SICU.

Cardiac Care Unit (CCU)

The *cardiac care unit (CCU)* is where adult patients with severe cardiac problems such as *acute myocardial infarction* (heart attack), cardiac arrest, or life-threatening *arrhythmias* (irregular heart rhythms) are taken care of. It is usually a cardiologist who heads up this unit and the interdisciplinary team, and it is run very similarly to the MICU and SICU in terms of nursing staff and layout. It also has the same monitoring capacity and ability to take care of patients on specialized machines such as a ventilator or an intra-aortic balloon pump (a machine used to help increase the output of the heart). In highly specialized hospitals, the CCU will be in addition to a CTU (see below) for cardiac patients who have had open heart or pulmonary surgery. Patients may initially be admitted to the CCU for a cardiac problem and then transferred to the CTU before or after heart surgery.

Cardiothoracic Care Unit (CTU)

The *cardiothoracic care unit (CTU)* specializes in caring for patients after cardiothoracic surgery or occasionally for very sick patients who will undergo such surgery. Examples of these surgeries include valve replacement, coronary artery bypass, and aortic repair. Cardiothoracic surgeons are usually the attending physicians in this unit, and there may be medical or surgical intensive care physicians to manage patient care as well with the interdisciplinary team of providers. Although heart surgeries are performed quite routinely these days, patients undergoing these operations require an enormous amount of specialized care immediately after surgery.

Neurosurgical Intensive Care Unit (NSCU or NSICU)

The *neurosurgical intensive care unit (NSCU* or *NSICU)* is where adult patients with severe brain or spinal cord injuries are taken care of. Patients will go to this unit after a neurosurgical operation or procedure for observation or for ongoing care. For example, if you had bleeding on the brain and it had to be drained, you would be placed in this unit. Other reasons for admission to this unit include epilepsy monitoring and care for a brain tumor. This unit is often run by a neurosurgeon or a neurologist. Staffing ratios and monitoring capabilities mirror that of the other ICUs.

Post-anesthesia Care Unit (PACU, Recovery Room)

The *post-anesthesia care unit (PACU)* is where you go right after surgery while you are still waking up from the anesthesia. Anesthesiologists supervise the staff in this unit. The nurses and medical providers need to make sure that you successfully come out of anesthesia and are able to breathe on your own. This is usually where family members are first allowed to lay eyes on their loved ones after surgery at the discretion of the doctor, nurses, PAs, and NPs, once the patient is stabilized. Although you may be drowsy or nauseated and may not remember much about receiving brief visits, it is usually very comforting for families and friends to spend time with you before you are transferred to your room. Although most patients are *recovered* in the PACU, for some types of surgeries and in specialized centers, you might be brought right to the ICU. This may also depend on how many beds and nurses are available in the PACU and also on the time of day that patients are emerging from surgery. For patients coming out of surgery after hours, the PACU may not be staffed to accommodate recovery. In this situation, patients may be recovered in the OR, or they will be taken to another monitored setting. Anesthesiologists and nurses will care for these patients while they wake up, regardless of the geographical location in the hospital.

Neonatal Intensive Care Unit (NICU)

The *neonatal intensive care unit (NICU)* is where newborn and premature babies are taken when they need extra care. Sometimes this is only for observation and sometimes for more serious conditions. Newborns with a mildly elevated *bilirubin* (a fluid produced by the liver) level may be admitted to the NICU for a few days. Sometimes babies are born with or acquire serious conditions such as a newborn fever or a heart or lung problem. Babies born with very low birth weight may not be able to feed or breathe on their own. These sick and tiny infants will require the specialized care of the highly trained neonatologists and neonatal nurses as well as the specialized equipment and machines found in the NICU. Whether the newborn's medical condition is not very serious or life-threatening, new parents and their families will find their child's admission to the NICU to be a stressful and worrisome time. Typically the NICU is staffed by individuals who are particularly sensitive and attuned to these circumstances.

Pediatric Intensive Care Unit (PICU)

The *pediatric intensive care unit (PICU)* is where infants through adolescents are taken care of for advanced or serious medical illnesses or injuries. The PICU and MICU take care of many similar medical illnesses; however, the PICU also admits children after serious surgeries. The PICU is run by pediatricians with advanced training in critical care—they are often referred to as pediatric intensivists. The nurses, PAs, and NPs who work in the PICU have had specialized or advanced training; enormous empathy as well as skill is required since taking care of gravely ill or injured children AND the needs of their parents is emotionally draining. Having a child admitted to the PICU is frightening; parents and families will need extra support. See chapter 12 for more information.

Burn Center

Only a limited number of hospitals have a specialized *burn center*. Taking care of full body burns requires not only special equipment such as a *hyperbaric chamber* (a space to treat certain conditions with oxygen therapy) but also highly trained specialists and nurses in wound care. These centers are needed not only for someone who has been burned in the traditional sense but also for someone with dangerous *dermatologic* (skin) conditions such as *Stevens Johnson syndrome* (severe blistering of the skin's top layer, typically brought on by a drug reaction). Anyone with a serious skin condition that is causing loss of skin is at serious risk of life-threatening fluid loss. If you fall into one of these categories and your present hospital does not have the capabilities, transfer will be made to another facility. Burn care is a highly specific medical subspecialty. If your family member is a burn patient, you must ensure that the proper care is rendered as this is critical to saving life and limb, literally. If you have any doubt about the quality of the care your loved one is receiving, speak with the doctors, nurses, and administrators. It is vitally important that patients with severe burns be cared for in a burn unit, even one that is far from home.

Tele-ICU (eICU, Electronic ICU)

As health care technology evolves, medical and surgical practitioners have found more innovative and creative ways to make use of it. In certain circumstances, it is not possible for nurses, physicians, and other health professionals to be on-site with patients requiring intensive medical care. This is where telemedicine comes into play. Telemedicine uses video equipment and telephones to allow experts to guide treatment remotely to the providers on-site with the

Tele-ICU as an Example of Tele-Health

In a true example of twenty-first-century health care, tele-ICU or eICU (e for electronic) has emerged as a method to care for patients in hospitals where either the patient cannot get to an ICU or the health professionals are unable to get to the hospital. The entire field is called tele-health or telemedicine, and you will continue to see huge growth in this area over the coming years. Whether it is smart phones, computers, video hookups, or social media, these methods have been put in place for improving and speeding up communication between the patient and the health care professional or between one health care professional and another. In the case of tele-ICU, the technology takes distance out of the equation, such that experts may offer consults remotely. This may sound like further depersonalization of modern medical care—and it may be—but it serves as a life-saving solution for certain situations.

patient. Geographically isolated hospitals and staffing shortages are two of the reasons that the *tele-ICU (eICU, electronic ICU)* has become popular. In addition, some hospitals prefer an extra layer of monitoring to improve early recognition of a change in a patient's condition. For example, since ICU patients require around-the-clock surveillance but there may not be enough nurses and doctors to be present in the hospital, patients can be watched via remote hook-ups so that care can be directed to the health professionals who are near the patients. Typically large urban centers have hospitals with ICUs and trained staff. If you are located in a rural or isolated area, your hospital may not have these capabilities. Telemedicine with audiovisual monitoring, computers, telephones, and highly trained doctors and nurses to guide treatment may mitigate these circumstances. Clearly, a telemedicine arrangement is wholly dependent on excellent communication and collaboration between health professionals.

Biocontainment Unit

In the recent era of highly dangerous and contagious infections such as Ebola and SARS, a few extremely specialized units have been constructed to both monitor patients and protect staff and visitors from contracting the disease. *Biocontainment units,* as they are known, are located within very sophisticated medical centers and require an extraordinary amount of money to maintain and to train health care professionals. They exist as a barrier to possible epidemics and are a hallmark of nations in which there are tremendous resources to combat diseases. If a patient with Ebola, for example, were to be detected at an airport or an ER, he or she would likely now be whisked away to a biocontainment unit.

Journey to the ICU

Henry came into the hospital for a little bout of pneumonia. They told him in the ER that since he was eighty-one years old, he was going to be admitted for some observation and IV antibiotics. The first day or two had gone well until Henry began having more trouble breathing. Nothing the doctors and nurses did seem to work. Now he was being transferred to the ICU, and people were talking about things he did not understand. Did he want a breathing tube? Did he want to be resuscitated? Was there someone they should call? Henry didn't remember anything after that, but his wife, Barbara, did. Barbara came right away after the hospital called. She wanted to rush in to see Henry, but the ICU has all these rules and she had to wait outside and could only visit for a short while. She did not understand all the medical terms and questions she was asked. What is a ventilator? What are pressors? Did Henry want to have CPR done on him? These are all questions Barbara did not know the answer to and wished someone would help her with. Fortunately, she felt comfortable with the daytime nurses, so she began to ask them questions.

ICU ORGANIZATION

The ICU attending physician—an *intensivist* usually employed by the hospital—is in charge of all the patients in the unit. Other doctors and health care professionals (such as specialists and the patient's primary medical doctor) are involved in the patient's care, but the intensivist leads the decision-making process. In other ICUs, the patient's own primary care doctor will organize care with consulting physicians in areas of concern. For example, if the patient has a known pulmonary doctor from the outside, who is trained in critical care, he or she can be the *attending of record* (doctor in charge) for that patient in the ICU.

TIP Why Your Own Doctor May Not Be Allowed to Take Care of You in the ICU

If you discover that your own doctors are not allowed to make decisions about patient care in the ICU, you will know that this is a closed ICU with the hospital intensivists in charge. The intensivists in charge will make every effort to consult your own doctors to make sure the best care is given and your past history and concerns are addressed.

STEPPING DOWN AND STEP-DOWN UNITS (INTERMEDIATE CARE UNITS)

Some hospitals have *step-down (intermediate care) units*. These areas are for patients who are judged no longer sick enough for the ICU but who need more medical attention than the regular floor can provide. This is very often seen in the days after a patient has had a stroke. Initially the patient may be critically ill and ICU-level attention is needed for things such as *TPA,* a clot-busting medication. After the initial critical period has passed, the patient still needs very close monitoring of vital signs, including blood pressure. This close observation may not be accomplished with the nurse-to-patient ratio on the general floor, so the patient is sent to a step-down unit for a few days before another transition to the general floor (ward). Patients will also often step down between ICU and general floors after open heart surgery and after weaning from mechanical ventilation. One feature of the step-down or intermediate care unit is that you may now be able to get out of bed after your stay in the ICU. This comes along with the good news that you, perhaps with some help, may be able to get to toilet facilities, as opposed to using bedpans or commodes. Many units are initiating very early physical therapy to accelerate recovery from critical illness.

CHAPTER 12

Special Patient Populations

Often patients with a particular condition or illness are *cohorted* (grouped together) and assigned to certain floors in the hospital because staff on these floors are trained to handle their special needs. There may also be physical aspects to the layout of the unit and specialized medical equipment to support these patients. Different populations of patients have different needs. This model of grouping them together improves efficiency and helps to ensure that the patient will get the best care possible. Small community hospitals will likely not have as many specialized units, whereas large academic medical centers will have more. Although many hospitals make efforts to keep certain types of patients together, the availability of a bed will influence the floor to which a patient is assigned. For critically ill patients, the various types of intensive care units (ICUs) serve their needs. If you or your family member falls into this category, please turn to chapter 11.

ONCOLOGY

Patients with cancer have specific sets of care needs; the cancer population is very diverse since there are many different kinds of cancer. Doctors will categorize cancer into *solid tumors* and *liquid tumors*. Solid tumors are cancers of the organs such as brain, breast, lung, pancreas, and colon. Liquid tumors are cancers that affect the bone marrow and are usually either lymphoma or leukemia. Standard treatments for cancer can include combinations of chemotherapy, radiation, and surgery.

These treatments, as well as the cancer itself, leave patients with a severely weakened immune system and put them at risk for contracting infections, some of which may be life-threatening. A common reason for the admission of an oncology patient is a *neutropenic* fever. This means that the patient has a fever that is dangerous because her or his treatment has reduced the white blood count so dramatically that the body cannot adequately fight infection.

Isolation

Many oncology patients contract communicable diseases *secondary* (as a consequence of and related to) to their weakened immune systems. Two such bacterial examples are a type of diarrhea called *C. diff.* and a skin infection caused by a superbug called *MRSA.* Superbugs are resistant to many types of antibiotics, which is why they are worrisome to doctors and scientists. When patients have a history of these infections, they will be placed on *isolation* to prevent the spread of illness to protect visitors and hospital staff. Sometimes isolation is in reverse and meant to protect the patients themselves and not the visitors. Visitors will be asked to wear protective garments such as a disposable gowns, gloves, and masks. Individuals who are ill should not visit an oncology patient since even something as simple as a cold virus puts cancer patients with compromised immune systems at risk.

TIP   *C. diff.*—Use Soap and Water, Not Alcohol-Based Gel

Although most germs will be killed by using the hand sanitizers you will see all over the hospital, the spores of the diarrhea-causing bacterium called *C. diff.* will not be killed. Therefore, if a patient is identified as having *C. diff.,* it is important to wash your hands with soap and water if you have had any contact with the patient or if you've been in the patient's room. *C. diff.* causes colitis (inflammation of the colon). The elderly and people who have other illnesses or conditions requiring prolonged antibiotics are more prone to getting *C. diff.* Cancer patients, because of their compromised immune systems, are extremely vulnerable to contracting this condition as a result of the effects of certain chemotherapy drugs.

Bone Marrow Transplant Unit

The bone marrow transplant unit treats some of the sickest oncology patients. Bone marrow is found inside your bones and is responsible for making all the different blood cells necessary for life, such as red blood cells, white blood cells, and platelets. In an attempt to treat certain blood cancers, patients will receive aggressive chemotherapy that essentially wipes out their immune systems so they can receive healthy bone marrow from a donor. Through a procedure, healthy individuals can donate bone marrow to an individual with cancer. The hope is that the healthy donor bone marrow will thrive in the recipient's body and make healthy instead of cancerous blood cells. Bone marrow transplant patients are highly susceptible to infection. You will not be able to visit a patient on this unit without first going through a specific protocol of washing and donning gowns, gloves, and masks.

When a patient who has had a highly communicable disease such as MRSA or *C. diff.* is transferred or discharged out of that room, there must be what is a called a ***terminal clean*** of the room. There are specific protocols and products that housekeeping personnel must use to kill and prevent the spread of these germs.

Food and Flowers on the Oncology Floor

You will notice that oncology floors have many rules; this is to keep the patients safe from contracting further illness. One of the rules is to not bring fresh fruit and flowers since food can harbor bacteria and fresh flowers can harbor fungi. Both bacteria and fungi can make someone with a weakened immune system very ill. If you feel the need to bring a gift of food, you should bring something that is commercially processed and packaged. Please avoid fresh and home-cooked food.

Visitors on the Oncology Floors

Visitors to the oncology floor will need to stop at the nursing station prior to visiting a patient. At the nursing station, you will find out what the specific rules and regulations are for the floor and whether you need to worry about isolation precautions. At the minimum, all visitors and hospital staff members must wash their hands before entering the room of an oncology patient. When oncology patients leave their rooms, particularly those who are neutropenic (having a low white blood cell count), they will wear masks to protect them from contracting an infection.

PATIENTS WITH COGNITIVE LOSS

Hospitals can be a very difficult and even dangerous place for patients with cognitive loss or dementia. When patients with these issues are taken out of their normal environment, they often become more confused and sometimes agitated. If your family member has dementia, make sure the staff knows whether confusion or agitation has occurred during previous hospital stays so that staff can anticipate and alter the environment to decrease problems. It is important to make sure these patients are placed near a window so they can distinguish between daytime and nighttime. It is also important to make sure they have their eyeglasses if they wear them at home, and hearing aids if they need them. During the daytime, it is also possible for the nurse to position the patient in a chair by the nursing station to keep a closer eye on him or her. Some hospitals have a large room for four or more patients with cognitive loss who need enhanced observation so that they can be kept safe. Some other hospitals also have *ACE (advanced care for elders)* units. These units use a multidisciplinary approach to help prevent the decline that elderly patients can have in the hospital. If your family member has dementia or displays confusion, be sure to ask to have him or her moved to an ACE unit if there is one and as appropriate to the patient's other medical needs.

DRUG AND ALCOHOL ABUSE

Unfortunately, sometimes the first time the doctors and hospital staff find out about a patient's drinking problem is when he or she starts to go through withdrawal. If someone drinks regularly and then comes to the hospital, where alcohol is not available, he or she may start to exhibit signs of withdrawal after about two days. These usually take the form of agitation, restlessness, and elevated heart rates and tremors. When this occurs, patients will be placed on a special protocol; they will be given a medication every few hours for a couple of days to prevent the symptoms of withdrawal. This process is called *detoxification*. If the withdrawal symptoms worsen and are difficult to control, the patient may be placed in the intensive care unit for closer observation.

A similar situation can happen with patients who are addicted to drugs. When they are without the drug, they go through withdrawal symptoms. These symptoms vary according to the drug used. For example, many people are addicted to pain medications such as opioids. When they are not given these in the hospital or they are given a dose lower than what their bodies are used to, they will have symptoms such as stomach pain, nausea, pupil dilation, and generally feeling very ill. These patients will be given medications to help with the withdrawal symptoms depending on the specific situation.

Many people smoke or chew tobacco despite the evidence that it is harmful. Some patients are able to manage giving up tobacco while in the hospital, but some cannot. Some people will feel jittery if they don't smoke for only a few hours. Patients who are suffering from tobacco withdrawal symptoms should alert the health provider so they can be prescribed a nicotine patch. The dose of the patch is determined by how many cigarettes are typically smoked per day.

RESPIRATORY CARE/VENTILATED PATIENTS

Some people have a *chronic* (ongoing and for a long period) need for the help of a ventilator, a machine that breathes for them. Most of these patients have a *tracheostomy* (a hole cut in the trachea, or windpipe, with a plastic tube inserted). With the tracheostomy in place, the ventilator can be hooked up to this tube. Taking care of patients on ventilators requires special training and often occurs in a respiratory care unit (also called a ventilator unit). Usually one of the doctors responsible for overseeing patients on ventilators is trained in pulmonary medicine; the nurses have extra training as well. Respiratory therapists are key personnel on these floors, since their specialty is precisely geared to caring for ventilated patients. This expertise is important because complications can arise; as an example, the tracheotomy tube may become dislodged. Patients on ventilators are at very high risk for contracting pneumonia; therefore, preventing this serious illness is a focus of care. Coming off the ventilator, called *weaning*, is frequently a goal for these patients and requires a carefully approached process by a multidisciplinary team. We discuss this process in chapter 11.

POSTSURGICAL INFECTIONS AND COMPLICATIONS

Not every surgery goes as planned. Complex surgeries requiring large incisions into the skin can make it difficult for the body to heal. This is particularly true in the setting of underlying medical conditions such as uncontrolled diabetes and the immunocompromised states found in patients on chronic steroids. Trained wound specialists must care for surgical wound infections. A dietitian also needs to be involved to ensure that the patient is receiving proper nutrition. Without the proper nutrients, the body cannot heal. If you have a wound complication, it is important to talk with the surgeons and wound care specialists (usually nurses) every day to understand the progress of the infection. Patients with poorly healing surgical wounds sometimes need to go back to the operating room.

STROKE PATIENTS/STROKE UNIT

After suffering a stroke (also known as a *cerebral vascular accident,* or *CVA*), patients require close monitoring. They need frequent checks of their neurologic functions as well as control of their blood pressure and other vital signs. Stroke units are designed to meet the special needs of post-stroke patients. These units take a multidisciplinary approach to post-stroke care to help patients regain functional status through physical and occupational therapy and also to prevent secondary complications of stroke such as infection, *aspiration*, and *deep vein thrombosis.*

PSYCHIATRIC PATIENTS

There are many different degrees and types of mental illness. Some people with psychiatric problems may come to the hospital for help with those conditions, while others may find that their conditions worsen once they are in the hospital. Psychiatrists, psychiatric nurses, and social workers will work with these patients to determine the best course of treatment for them.

Many patients with psychiatric conditions can be managed with the medical team on the medical floors. Some patients, however, will need a more controlled environment such as a psychiatric unit, which is usually a locked-down unit. Special access is required to get on and off these units. Medical doctors visit these patients to help continue treatment of other medical issues. Visitors are usually restricted to certain times a day. Psychiatric units are different from regular medical and surgery floors in that many patients have the leeway to walk around and go to a recreational area or an eating area. The bed layout may be set up dormitory style.

YOUR HOSPITALIZED CHILD

There is nothing more frightening than having your child be a patient in the hospital. Sometimes this happens all of sudden, and sometimes you will have time to prepare, as occurs with a scheduled surgery or cancer treatments. There are whole books dedicated to pediatric hospital stays, so we will be brief here. The most important thing is to try to make your child as comfortable and unafraid as possible. It will be helpful to bring items from home that you know will provide comfort to your child. For a small child it might be a favorite pillow or stuffed animal. For an older child it might be an iPod, iPad, or books and magazines. If the hospital stay is planned beforehand and if your child is old enough and understands, involve him or her in the packing. Pediatric floors are equipped to allow a parent to stay overnight, so when packing for a child, do not forget to pack for yourself and for what YOU need to be comfortable as well. Just as you would pack for a trip, make a list so that you do not forget important things.

These days, social media are a great way for you and your child to stay connected with the outside world. They allow parents, other children, extended family, and friends to keep in touch with one another. For children with conditions commonly requiring hospitalization, social media may also provide a way to get peer encouragement from online support groups.

Having a child in the hospital is anxiety-producing, stressful, and frightening for parents and other family members. Many parents feel ill equipped to answer their child's questions about illnesses, treatment, and pain. However, most hospitals have supportive services in place to help you realize that you are not in this alone. Pediatric floors are staffed with many types of trained specialists to help you navigate every step of a pediatric inpatient stay. A *child life advocate* is one of these trained specialists. He or she has many tools and strategies through art or play to help children sort through feelings. Social workers and psychologists may provide additional support. Of course, the kind of individual who pursues a career in pediatric nursing will also have the skills to help children cope.

Although pediatric hospitalization is not the focus here, you may find that the information in many other chapters is helpful in navigating your child's inpatient stay.

General Pediatric Floors

Depending on the nature of your child's illness, he or she may be on a general pediatric floor or one that specializes in the care of serious illnesses and injuries. In addition to pediatric units, large, complex medical centers may also have an adolescent unit to serve the unique needs of patients in their teens.

NICU

The *neonatal intensive care unit* (*NICU*) is where newborn and premature babies are taken care of when they need to be observed or when they have conditions that are more serious. Babies born with very low birth weight may not be able to feed or breathe on their own. These sick and tiny infants will require the specialized care of highly trained neonatologists and neonatal nurses, as well as the specialized equipment and machines found in the NICU. Even if the newborn's medical condition is not likely to be life threatening such as in the case of elevated bilirubin (a fluid made in the liver), new parents and their families will find their child's admission to the NICU to be a stressful and worrisome time. Typically, the NICU is staffed by individuals who are particularly sensitive to parental anxieties and concerns.

PICU

The *pediatric intensive care unit* (*PICU*) is where infants through adolescents are taken care of for advanced or serious medical illnesses or injuries and after long, complex surgeries. The PICU is run by pediatricians with advanced training in critical care; they are often referred to as pediatric intensivists. The nurses, PAs, and NPs who work in the PICU have had specialized advanced training. Enormous empathy as well as skill is required to care for gravely ill or injured children and to attend to the needs of their parents. Having a child admitted to the PICU is frightening; parents and families will need extra support. The child life specialists will be instrumental in this regard.

OBSTETRICAL (OB) PATIENTS

For women expecting and planning to deliver in the hospital, there is usually plenty of time to plan for the stay or even to anticipate an early delivery. Since this topic has been extensively covered in many fine and thorough books, we will not attempt to address general obstetric admissions in detail. Unlike some of the other floors in the hospital, the maternity ward is a happy place with families celebrating the birth of a new baby. After giving birth, mothers will stay in the hospital briefly (a couple of days typically) for a vaginal delivery and a little longer for a cesarean section. (Some women may not realize that a cesarean section is abdominal surgery that requires significant healing.) All hospitalized patients, including women in labor, will receive an IV in case medications need to be given, and the IV will likely stay in place until discharge. As with protocols on all the other medical and surgical floors, nurses will come to check on obstetrical patients a few times during their shift to monitor vital signs (blood pressure, heart rate, respiratory rate, and temperature). If you came from home with regular medications, you will be given them in the hospital as long as they are approved by your doctor. During the stay, obstetrical patients may be prescribed some additional medications; among the most common are pain medications. These can be something benign, such as ibuprofen, or something stronger, such as an opioid. If you are on opioids—which are commonly given after cesarean section—you will likely be on a stool softener as well. You will be advised to get up and walk around as soon as possible since the sooner you are back on your feet, the better you will feel.

TIP Medications for Pregnant and Nursing Mothers

As we have advised for all other types of patients, if you have questions about any aspect of care or medication, be sure to ask your health care team. Pregnant women who are hospitalized prior to delivery will want to exercise extreme vigilance about medications prescribed, particularly if the providers are not trained in obstetrics. Many commonly prescribed—including over-the-counter—medications may be harmful for the fetus. Nursing mothers will have concerns about what medications pass through the breast milk to the infant.

There are other scenarios in which pregnant women may be hospitalized prior to delivery. If the pregnancy poses a threat to the fetus or mother, if preterm labor compromises the pregnancy, or if a complicated multiple birth is anticipated, a woman may be admitted for several weeks before the due date. Occasionally, there is a sad outcome from a pregnancy. Examples include *fetal demise* (stillbirth) or very compromised babies not expected to survive. In this case, it will be particularly difficult for you as the mother to be surrounded by glowing new parents with healthy newborns in nearby rooms. In some hospitals, you will be moved to a quiet corner or away from the general obstetric floor. Should you be in this unfortunate circumstance and if it would help with coping, you should ask to be moved away from the maternity unit.

What's This For???

Sometimes nurses take for granted that patients will know or understand something they find commonplace. When I gave birth to my first child, I was a second-year medical resident. After the delivery while in the recovery area, I was sent to use the bathroom armed with a small plastic bottle with a spout. I went into the bathroom, stared at that bottle, and honestly had no idea what I was supposed to do with it. I wasn't sure if they thought I knew because I was a doctor or if this was something everyone was supposed to know. I finally summoned enough courage to come out of the bathroom and find the nurse to ask her what I was supposed to do with the bottle. Turns out it was a *peribottle,* which you are supposed to use after delivery to spray your bottom with warm water in place of toilet paper. Who knew??—*Karen Friedman*

In addition to childbirth, there are some other scenarios for obstetrical patients. A pregnant woman may find herself hospitalized for a reason that has nothing to do with her pregnancy, such as pneumonia or a gallbladder issue. When this occurs, she will often be placed on the general medical floors. If you find yourself in this situation, it is extra important to be vigilant with the physicians, particularly physicians in training. Do not hesitate to question the doctors about any new medication that is prescribed. Ask them if they know about the safety profile of the medication for pregnant females. Even what may seem to be benign over-the- counter medications have the potential to be harmful in pregnancy. One example is ibuprofen; many people take it routinely for headaches, muscle soreness, and pain. However, **ibuprofen is not considered safe during pregnancy as it poses risks to the unborn baby.** The Internet is full of lists of medications that are safe in pregnancy. If you are pregnant, we urge you to perform due diligence in researching the safety profile of any medications prescribed during this vulnerable time.

EXTENDED STAYS

Some patients end up staying in the hospital for a long period as a consequence of their illness or injury. When this occurs, it tends to be very burdensome—emotionally and financially—for the patient's family and friends. Family members will set up a rotating schedule so that someone can be present when the patient is undergoing important tests and procedures or can help with communicating with health care professionals. It is sometimes possible to stay by a family member's bedside overnight; often hospitals will have chairs that fold out into a bed. Many hospitals also have other amenities for families with long-stay patients, such as parking vouchers and complimentary meals. You will need to do some investigating to discover what is available. Nursing staff, nurse managers, and the unit clerks may be helpful in this regard. Do not hesitate to inquire about the options.

CLINICAL TRIALS

How do researchers figure out if medications or procedures are effective and safe? In the United States, there is a lengthy process overseen by the *Food and Drug Administration* (FDA) to determine whether medications can be marketed without causing undue harm. Typically, after medications are developed in the laboratory, they are tested on animals, then on small groups of human volunteers. Many medications do not make it past this stage. However, those drugs that do get to this stage must then be tested on large groups of people to see if they are safe and effective in the real-world setting, where there are all types of variability. Particularly in academic medical centers, testing new medications is extremely common. If you have a certain illness or condition, you may be approached by a *clinical research coordinator* or *research nurse* to see if you fit criteria to participate in a study to test a drug. In addition to the control of the FDA, there are hospital organizations that ensure safety for patients participating in such research. Most of the time a new, experimental drug is tested in two or more groups of similar patients against either a *placebo* (fake drug) or a known alternative medication. In a process called randomization, a computer chooses which group the participant is entered into. You will not be able to choose your group, nor will you know if you are getting the new drug. If neither you nor the research team knows which group you are in, this is called a double-blind study, and it is considered the most rigorous type of study. However, there are all types of drug studies, and sometimes only the experimental drug is tested without a comparison group. In this case, the doctors, nurses, and patients are aware of the treatment. If you decide to be in a study, you will be helping science. Although it is not guaranteed, you may derive some direct benefit, and certainly you will have a little more medical scrutiny since the research team is very interested in the effects of the treatment. We know from media reports, however, that there are situations in which drugs previously thought to be safe turn out to have serious side effects. Only you can decide whether you want to be involved in this type of research.

ADVANCE DIRECTIVES

A hospital episode is not really the right time to decide what you want done should something catastrophic occur (heart or breathing stops, brain function is compromised). These conversations should ideally take place at home with your loved ones when you are in a state of reasonable health and when your emotional state is not challenged. Alternatively, this conversation can take place in a primary care provider's office or with a surgeon or other specialist before a planned hospitalization, although not all physicians have the training to hold these discussions.

Unfortunately, many individuals do not confront these difficult questions until during an inpatient stay, when they are asked to designate their preferences. As a result, discussions about advance directives are too often held at the last possible moment in the worst possible circumstances. When patients are able to understand information and make decisions for

Clinical Trial Process

Here is the process:

You will be informed about the nature of the clinical trial and the drugs or devices involved.
You will be asked to sign a consent form and to ask as many questions as you wish.
You will be instructed that you can change your mind if you no longer to wish to remain in the study.
You will be given telephone numbers and individuals to contact if you have questions or problems.
You will be given a list of possible risks (but also benefits).
You will be told exactly what you will be expected to do to be in the study (take medication, fill out surveys, return for office visits, respond to telephone calls, fill out pill diaries).

Remember that the decision to participate is completely up to you.

themselves, nurses may ask about their wishes should their hearts stop. The question might be posed as, "Do you want to be **resuscitated**?" Resuscitation means the doctor will shock your heart if it stops beating or will put a plastic tube down your throat (**intubation**) and hook you up to a ventilator if you stop breathing. These measures are an attempt to bring you back to life, although many times they fail to accomplish the intent.

If something serious happens in the hospital and you cannot make these decisions, the doctors and nurses will ask your **health care proxy** (an individual entrusted to make medical decisions for another individual). It is therefore vitally important to designate a health care proxy. This is someone who knows your wishes and can act on your behalf when it is necessary to make these critical medical decisions. If there is no health care proxy appointed, the decisions go to the next of kin. These are hard decisions to make; careful thought and attention must be given. Sadly, when family members have not received information about loved ones' wishes and preferences about resuscitation, there may be dissent and discord. For this reason, to spare loved ones from these conflicts, it is best to anticipate responses to these difficult questions by preparing an **advance directive**, a document outlining what the patient wants done in life-threatening emergencies.

Medical illness or traumatic injury can be a time of tremendous family stress. Even the most functional of families can become distressed and confused when faced with life-or-death decisions. This is why it is so important to have conversations before becoming ill and to have a health care proxy and a **living will** (one form of advance directive) designated. When a family member is incapacitated and there is neither a health care proxy nor an official next of kin (for example, the spouse is deceased), the children are left with the burden of decision making. If there are many children, there may be differences of opinions and personalities that make coming to a consensus very difficult.

ETHICS COMMITTEES

Moral and ethical dilemmas can arise in the course of patient care. Sometimes family members will interfere with a patient's known wishes or will try to prevent physicians from disclosing important information to a patient. Many hospitals have *ethics committees* set up to assist families, patients, and the health care professionals involved in these situations. These committees will give guidance to help make decisions grounded in sound ethical practices. In cases when there are difficult questions—for example, a person's religion is in conflict with state law or hospital policy—a legal professional can be called in to help.

TIP   Family Consensus and Communication with Providers

When making decisions for a loved one who has not expressed clear wishes about medical treatment, consensus among family members can be a painful and emotional time. This may be further complicated by the need to gather information from the providers and to relay choices about how much intervention is desired. If possible, families should pick a designated person to communicate with the health care team. It is both time-intensive and confusing for the health care team if different family members are contacting them at different times and with different demands.

THE END OF LIFE

Palliative Care

Many people come to the hospital with devastating medical illness or injury. For these individuals, end-of-life issues will need to be addressed. Thankfully, our health care systems have come a long way in the United States, and we have begun to value the preservation of quality of life, time with family, and pain relief over preservation of life at any cost to the patient and families. Many hospitals have well-defined *palliative care* teams to help families and health care providers deal with end-of-life issues. These teams are interdisciplinary and are usually made up of physicians, nurse practitioners, physician assistants, nurses, social workers, and case managers. Palliative care medicine is now a recognized fellowship that requires a physician to have additional years of training, which includes advanced knowledge of pain control and advanced communication skills. These skills are most essential for conversations about *goals of care* with families. These conversations explore the status of the medical illness, provide a realistic appraisal of what may happen to the patient, and explore the existing end-of-life objectives. The palliative care team's extra training allows them to aid in the emotional and physical pain of end-of-life situations.

End-of-life decisions are very personal, requiring a great deal of input from patients and families. Some patients and families want everything done at all costs to preserve life, while others see the end of life as inevitable and simply want comfort measures, with others falling in between those extremes. The palliative care team is often asked to shoulder the responsibility of end-of-life pain management, with the guiding principle that no patient should ever suffer regardless of what the goals of care are. For patients on a palliative service, pain management is always available and is encouraged for patients who are suffering. When the goals of care become *comfort measures*—meaning no further testing, workup, or treatment is wanted—it may be appropriate to transfer patients off the medical floors and move them to another area of the hospital called a palliative care unit. These units have larger private rooms to accommodate family visiting.

Hospice

Patients on palliative care can be transitioned to hospice care. *Hospice* is a service provided through insurance, usually Medicare, that allows a patient to be *palliated* (cared for with comfort measures) in a facility such as a hospital or nursing home or at home. Most patients will go home on hospice care if their life expectancy is a few weeks to a few months. Patients will go on inpatient hospice when the life expectancy can be counted in days. If you or your family member is eligible for hospice, you will be seen by a hospice representative who can explain the benefit. Hospice provides on-site care for only about four hours a day depending on the situation. This means that if you or your family member requires around-the-clock care—for example, help with toileting, dressing, or walking—you will need to hire a private aide to perform these duties. However, hospice does provide around-the-clock support with nurses and physicians on hand to help deal with symptom management and medication changes and to make home visits as needed.

CHAPTER 13

Elective Surgery

EVOLUTION OF SURGERY

The science of surgery has evolved significantly over the past fifty years. It may seem miraculous to older individuals that the conditions that used to signal certain demise can now be repaired surgically. Think about blocked coronary arteries: prior to the 1960s, who could have predicted that a heart could be restored or blood vessels propped open, with patients going home four days after surgery?

Or consider how many people you know who have been able to walk comfortably and even play sports after knee and hip replacements.

In the past fifteen years, the most common surgeries requiring an in-patient stay include knee and hip replacement, spinal surgery, *cholecystectomy* (gallbladder removal), and cesarean section. If you require *elective* (planned) surgery, your doctor will determine if it can safely be performed as *ambulatory* (outpatient) surgery or if you need to be admitted to the hospital.

MINIMALLY INVASIVE VERSUS OPEN SURGERY

Many surgeries that used to be performed as "open," which means cutting through the skin, can now be performed *laparoscopically* (by the creation of tiny holes through which instruments are inserted into the abdomen and then controlled by the surgeon). When the instruments are inserted into the chest, the procedure is called *thorascopic* surgery. These surgeries are also referred to as minimally invasive. The increasing popularity of laparoscopic techniques has drastically cut down on time in the hospital. In fact, as a result of advances in technology and anesthesiology, there is a trend for *gynecologic* (pertaining to female reproductive organs) surgery and gall bladder removal to be performed in an outpatient setting. Nonetheless, patients do often spend a night or two in the hospital after many types of surgery, even minimally invasive, with the patient's underlying preoperative condition being one of the determining factors. The length of stay (LOS), as it is called in the hospital, depends on the type of anesthesia, risk of bleeding, the patient's ability to get out of bed, and whether there are postoperative complications.

UNPLANNED VERSUS ELECTIVE SURGERY

There is an enormous difference in preparation processes between unplanned and elective surgeries. If you have entered the hospital through the emergency room or if you are already in the hospital and it is determined that you need surgery, you will not have time to prepare, mentally, physically, or emotionally. In this chapter, we will outline the experience of navigating the stay for a planned surgery. We will discuss the before, during, and after of an inpatient surgical stay.

PLANNING FOR SURGERY

Visitors

If you know you will be spending some time in the hospital, whether it is for a day or many more, you will have time to prepare. You will have time to pack a bag with books, music, clothes, and favorite toiletries. You can let your friends and family members know that you will be out of the loop for a time and can express your preference about visitors. Having visitors is a very personal and individualized matter. Some people like to be left alone to recover in peace, while others enjoy the distraction and are pleased to see loved ones right away. Recent evidence suggests that having friends or family spend the day visiting with you improves recovery. Most hospitals will now permit family members to stay overnight to support their loved one. Remember that you won't be looking and feeling your best for a day or two after the operation, so it is important to think about the specific visitors who you know will bring you comfort. This may be someone who will provide a calming presence or has a good sense of what your needs will be—someone, for instance, who can find you an extra pillow and provide help sitting up or getting the nurse's attention if you are in pain. The right visitor can be a superb advocate for you when you most need it.

TIP   Visitors after Surgery

Remember that it is not your job to entertain visitors or assure them that you will be fine. The downside of having visitors after surgery is that you may not look or feel terrific. You may have pain or nausea. You may not be able to get out of bed immediately and will need to use a bedpan or commode. Having many visitors may initially feel intrusive. Take care of yourself first. Visits from nonessential family and friends can take place later, or at home. Visitors may mean well but can be distressing, noisy, and nosy. Before you invite friends and family to see you in the hospital, think carefully about who will bring you comfort or distraction.

Getting Ready for Surgery (Optimization)/Pre-Op Counseling

If you have a few months in which to prepare for surgery, you may be advised to lose weight, stop smoking, or get better control of your diabetes. If you are underweight or have nutritional deficiencies, you may be advised to eat certain foods or take supplements to boost your nutritional status. Medical professionals term these healthful preparation processes *optimization*. We now know, through scores of research studies, that patients have better outcomes after surgery if they are as healthy and strong as possible before surgery. Older patients in particular are at risk for deconditioning after only a few days in the hospital. Therefore, eating well and exercising before the operation may mean feeling better afterward.

The surgeon's office will provide you with written instructions about how best to prepare for your operation. Indeed, you will also get advice from everyone from the surgical scheduler (not a medical professional) to the surgeon. Please take advantage of the opportunity to discuss how you can best prepare for surgery. The nurse or nurse practitioner in the office may be the best source of information.

Optimization before Joint Replacement

Patients who will undergo *joint arthroplasty* (joint replacement) surgery involving insertion of *prosthetic* (artificial) knees, hips, or shoulder joints will typically have quite a while to get themselves into shape. There are some surgeons who will not operate on patients to replace a knee or hip until the patient has stopped smoking, gotten below a certain weight, or has better control of his or her diabetes. This is because surgeons now know that patients have more complications after these types of surgery if they go into it with these factors.

TIP Advice to Prepare for Surgery and Finding the Right Surgeon

If you do not feel you are getting good advice on how to prepare for your surgery and your requests remain unanswered, it might be time to pick another surgeon. Preparing for your surgery is a very important part of the process and influences the outcome and the recovery process, so don't neglect this important step.

Dental Work and Oral Hygiene before Surgery

If you will have general anesthesia and will need *endotracheal tube* insertion through the mouth into the *trachea* (windpipe), you may be advised before surgery to have loose teeth pulled or to have a good dental cleaning. To protect you, surgeons and anesthesiologists, devoted to first doing no harm, want to make sure that you come to surgery with a healthy mouth, which in turn will ensure a better outcome. Therefore, prior to surgery, you may be advised to use special rinses and adopt a tooth-brushing routine to rid the mouth area of bacteria. This will be especially important in the twenty-four hours before surgery since anesthesia is introduced through a tube in the mouth.

Presurgical Testing and Clearance

You and your doctor have decided you need surgery. The riskiest part of most surgeries is undergoing anesthesia, which is like having a stress test on your heart. The doctor will want to make sure you—in particular, your heart and lungs—are at your best before you go under anesthesia. This is called *medical optimization*. Every time you need surgery, the risks and benefits must be evaluated. The doctors and nurses will ask a series of questions to help determine if you need testing prior to your operation. One of the things they are trying to determine is your *METS,* or *metabolic equivalents.* How much exercise can you tolerate? Can you walk only a few steps, or are you able to run to catch the bus? On the basis of the information gathered, you may or may not need prior testing before the planned surgery. Some examples of these tests are: *stress test, angiogram (cardiac catheterization), echocardiogram* (sonogram of the heart), and *pulmonary function tests* (breathing tests). These tests are explained in chapter 8. If your surgery is urgent, there is no time for presurgical testing and you go straight to surgery. We discuss this in chapter 14.

Antibiotic Prophylaxis

Depending on the type of surgery you will have, you may be given an antibiotic before surgery to prevent infection. This is because surgery can put you at risk for infections. This is particularly true if the surgical procedure you are having involves placing a foreign object inside your body. Some common examples of foreign objects are pacemakers, artificial valves, and artificial joints. Because of the risk of infection resulting from these operations, the doctor may recommend *prophylactic* (preventive) antibiotics. These are antibiotics that will be given in the *perioperative* period, right before and for a short time after surgery. The doses, types, and duration of the antibiotic medication vary for the type of operation and the preoperative medical status of the patient.

NPO

As previously discussed, *NPO* stands for the Latin phrase *non per os,* meaning nothing per mouth. If you are scheduled for surgery, there will be no eating or drinking for at least six hours before the operation. If you vomit with food in the stomach while under anesthesia, you run the risk of getting *aspiration* pneumonia. It is extremely important that if you are told not to take any food or drink, you comply with this instruction. Patients are usually allowed to take their daily medications with a sip of water, however.

Shared Decision Making

Fortunately, in recent years the medical field has moved away from a paternalistic approach, which put physicians at the top of the hierarchy, with patients at the bottom, who were expected to follow directions without questioning the doctor's reasons and rationale. When it comes to choosing between treatment options, it is important for patients to express their own wishes. Elective surgery is a prime example. Shared decision making involves collaboration between providers and patients, allowing both parties to reach a consensus about treatment, using available medical information and taking into consideration the patient's preferences and values.

TIP   Medications on Day of Elective Surgery

Ask your doctor to clarify which medications are approved before surgery and which must be avoided. Confirm whether a sip of water is permitted on the morning of your surgery to take your medications.

Same-Day Admit

Same-day admit means that you will not spend the night before surgery in the hospital. You will be given a time to report to the hospital, which will depend on where you are on the surgeon's list of cases for the day. You will be asked to change into a hospital gown, cap, and booties. The anesthesiologist will visit you to make sure you are ready for surgery by speaking with you and by reviewing the notes from the presurgical clearance team. The anesthesiologist will ask you again if you have eaten or had anything to drink. Your risks of anesthesia will be explained, and you will be asked to sign consent to have anesthesia administered. Either before or after the anesthesiologist sees you, the surgeon will visit you to go over your surgery and will obtain consent. In most hospitals, the surgeon will mark your skin with a special pen to designate where the operation will occur and will sign with his or her initials. If you are in a teaching hospital, the surgeon will be accompanied by *residents*, *fellows*, and students. You may also meet physician assistants specially trained in surgical techniques. Typically surgeons work with the same PAs over and over again

The Schedule and the Waiting Room

One of the most frustrating things that patients and families experience is delays with a scheduled surgery. Waiting for an operation is usually a tense period; the patient is hungry and thirsty, and family and friends are nervously waiting in a cramped, curtained-off area that offers little privacy and no comfort or calm. Even though the surgery was scheduled for 7:30 a.m. and it is now 9:00 a.m., no one has stopped by to update anyone about when the surgery will actually occur. What might have happened?

Here are some possibilities:

During early morning rounds, the surgical team discovered that another patient had a complication requiring immediate attention.

There is a wait for the operating room to be cleaned.

The surgical instruments were not prepared.

The surgeon had trouble getting his or her kids out the door to day care.

You get the picture.

Now imagine that you are the surgeon's third case on the schedule—EVERY effort to create a smooth process is such that their communications and procedures are exquisitely orchestrated. This is different from the teaching that occurs with residents, fellows, and students. The PA is a full participant in the surgery and knows exactly what to do while working in concert with the surgical team.

defeated. Even worse than delays before leaving the same-day admitting area are the ones when the patient has been wheeled to the operating room and the delay happens just prior to surgery. More often than not, the duration of surgery goes as expected, but the hidden delay to start time is responsible for a longer-than-anticipated waiting period.

TIP Marking the Site of Surgery

Always ask your surgeon to put his or her initials where he or she is going to operate. This is a safety measure to help ensure that the exact place you have discussed having the operation is precisely where it will occur. Many hospitals require this practice. However, if they do not, it is your job to insist by asking the surgeon to mark the spot and personalize it.

TIP Updates about Patients Undergoing Surgery

If you are told to expect a four-hour surgery but it begins two hours late, it can be a frightening time for families in the waiting room. Make sure that you clearly explain to staff that you want updates about how the operation is proceeding and when it might be expected to finish. Some hospitals are using pagers to keep families in the loop. Sometimes a nurse will pop out of the OR (operating room) to update the family. Ask when exactly the operation started or when anesthesia was *induced*. After anesthesia, add another thirty to forty-five minutes for the time it takes to prepare, drape (with sterile cloths), and position the patient before the surgeon starts.

AFTER SURGERY

Post-anesthesia Care Unit (PACU, Recovery Room)

The *post-anesthesia care unit (PACU)* is where patients go right after surgery while they are still waking up from the anesthesia. Anesthesiologists care for patients in this unit. The nurses need to make sure that you successfully come out of anesthesia and are able to breathe on your own. This is usually where family members are first allowed to lay eyes on their loved ones after surgery at the discretion of the doctor, nurses, PAs, and NPs once the patient is stabilized. Although patients may be drowsy or nauseated and may not remember much about receiving brief visits, it is usually very comforting for families and friends to spend a moment with their loved one or to stay and hold their loved one's hand before he or she is transferred to the unit. On occasion, following certain surgical procedures, the patient might be brought directly from the OR to the ICU by the anesthesiologist. For example, in a medical center with a specialized cardiothoracic unit, the team (consisting of surgeons, nurses, PAs, and intensivists) will need to monitor the patient in their own specialized setting. Recovery location may also depend on how many spaces and nurses are available in the PACU and also on the time of day that patients are emerging from surgery. If you end up being the last case of the day and surgery ends after typical hours, the PACU may not be adequately staffed to manage patients coming out of surgery. In this case, recovery from anesthesia may occur on the surgical floor or ICU but under the supervision of trained staff.

Getting Settled in Your Room after Surgery

If you are a same-day admit patient, then you will not have seen your room until after surgery. Depending on the type of hospital, you may be on a unit (and of course, in a room) with other surgery patients. Some hospitals have a mixed *med-surg* (medical and surgical) unit where both types of patients are placed. More specialized and larger medical centers will have units for surgical patients only. The health care professionals taking care of you on specialized units—nursing staff, nurse practitioners, physician assistants, patient care associates, physical therapists, and discharge planners—have expertise in caring for patients with exactly the types of conditions that you will have after surgery.

Contact with the Surgical Team after Surgery

At least once a day, someone from the surgical team will *round* (come to see you) to check the dressing and drains and will make sure that the *surgical wound* (where the incision was made) is healing well. In addition to these rounds, the nurse will contact the surgeon if there are any concerns about the wound or your general recovery. Many recovery processes after surgery occur by predetermined protocols—as soon as the patient achieves a certain milestone, the next step in the process can occur. For example, on the first postoperative day, you will be encouraged to stand up and shuffle to a chair. This will set you up for a short walk around your room later that day or the following day. In a similar fashion, your diet and pain control will also move through stages as you progress toward normalcy.

Pain Control

Patients who have undergone an operation will typically experience pain afterward. As you can imagine—particularly with "open" procedures in which incisions are made through skin, muscle, and bone—this pain can be quite severe. Many things influence patients' experience of pain. Males and females display tolerance differently, personality plays a key role, and even ethnicity and culture influence pain tolerance. Huge advances in anesthetic techniques and medications have changed the experience of pain after surgery.

Pain Medications
If you listen to the news or read the newspaper, you will know that opioid overuse and abuse has become an epic problem in the United States. Therefore, there is increasing effort to find nonnarcotic approaches to dealing with pain. Many research studies are currently being conducted to discover "opioid-sparing" methods to reduce pain. The type and location of anesthesia are examples. Giving nonnarcotic medications such as *NSAIDs (ibuprofen and naproxen sodium)* and *acetaminophen* during

the surgery is also being tested. The goal is to prevent the onset of pain and to block the pain receptors before the pain begins. Depending on the type of surgery, the anesthesiologist may administer a nerve block in the operating room to control your pain and to prevent the need for pain medication.

Patient-Controlled Analgesia (PCA)

After surgery, many patients will be able to "order" their own pain medication through a *PCA*, which is a **patient-controlled analgesia** pump. Pain medication, typically narcotics, is delivered to the blood through the IV when the patient pushes a button. To prevent overdose, timing and dosage limits are preset. Sometimes, patients experience extreme pain even when the PCA is delivering medication. If you are really miserable, it is important to let the nurse and other health care professionals know about it. Everyone has different pain medication needs and requires different doses of pain medication. It is important to make the hospital staff aware that you are in pain so they can adjust the dose or even change the medication.

DVT Prophylaxis

Here is a paradox: if you are on a blood thinner or aspirin before surgery, you will likely be asked to stop taking it a few days before your scheduled surgery. Too much bleeding during an operation is unsafe. However, there are certain surgical procedures that put patients at risk for developing blood clots—common ones include hip and knee replacement, as well as cardiac and abdominal surgery. Therefore, soon after surgery and after the bleeding has slowed down or stopped, it is likely that you will either be put back on a blood thinner or aspirin or be started on one of these medications to prevent **venous thromboembolism** (blood clots).

A clot results when the blood is not flowing well. Often clots form in the legs, where people may or may not experience symptoms (pain, swelling, redness, tenderness). This is called a **deep vein thrombosis (DVT)**. The real danger exists when a clot travels from the legs or the arms to the lung. This is called a **pulmonary embolism (PE)**. If this occurs, you may experience pain in your chest or difficulty breathing. Very rarely it can cause sudden death. After surgery, you will be prescribed injections or pills of **anticoagulant** (blood-thinning) medication to prevent clots. You may also be put on *sequential compression devices (Venodynes),* either with or without anticoagulant medication. While you are in bed, these devices surround your leg and periodically compress your legs to keep the blood flowing well. There are also *TEDS (compression stockings)* that can be worn when you are not in the bed. If you are able to walk, and if you are encouraged by your doctor to do so, vigorous and constant walking will also help to reduce your risk of clots.

Diet after Surgery

Depending on the type of surgery and what organs and body parts are affected, food will be gradually reintroduced after your surgery. If there has been a very major operation, particularly if any of the digestive organs have been operated on, the reintroduction may be very gradual. Often after surgery involving the bowels, the doctors and nurses will check you daily to see whether you are making bowel sounds again and passing gas. These signs indicate that the bowel is functioning again and ready for the reintroduction of food. During this time, the doctors and nurses will evaluate whether your digestive tract is ready for more of a challenge. You might start with clear liquids and ices and then move to solid foods as the staff determines that your digestive tract is working normally. It could be several days until you are ready for a normal diet. A major complication after surgery is *postoperative ileus.* This is a condition in which the bowel slows down so much that it is as if there is a *mechanical obstruction* (blockage). When this occurs, your belly will become severely distended; you can become nauseated and vomit. If there is a postoperative ileus, there may be a need to place an *NG* tube for decompression. As in all things, any questions should be directed to your nurse or your health care provider.

Rehab versus Home

The question of whether you will be sent to a rehabilitation facility (also called a subacute facility or a *skilled nursing facility*) is dependent on many factors and is part of a changing medical landscape due to insurance and government payers (Medicare and Medicaid), regulations, and compensation. In addition, there are regional differences in where patients go after the hospital. In short, we are unable to predict or generalize whether you will return to your previous living arrangement directly after the hospital stay since there are so many factors involved. For surgery patients, the discharge disposition considerations include the physical layout of the home environment (such as stairs), whether your muscles have to be retrained by experts (physical and occupational therapy), and your baseline health status. Generally, and as we would expect, a younger, previously healthy person will need fewer services after discharge, and an older, sicker patient will need more.

Finding out the best possible match between the patient and the rehab center is the job of the case managers. These trained professionals might begin making phone calls to facilities the moment you arrive at the hospital. It is important that you and your family members participate in the identification and location of the facility to which you will be discharged if you are not returning home. Ideally the facility should be close to where your family and friends can visit regularly. In contrast to emergency surgery or medical hospitalization, your health professional team usually can determine prior to surgery where you are most likely to be placed, taking into consideration all your baseline characteristics, the type of surgery, and the usual postoperative trajectory. However, sometimes complications occur or another condition reveals itself, and patients who expect to go home are safer and better served by going to a subacute rehab facility prior to returning home. We discuss many more details about discharge planning and suitability of discharge to home rather than a rehab facility in chapter 15.

CONVERTING FROM AMBULATORY (OUTPATIENT) SURGERY TO ADMISSION

Increasingly, many operations that were previously performed in the hospital are now taking place in ambulatory surgery centers (ASC) or surgicenters. If you have planned to have your surgery in a surgicenter, then it is likely that you are not reading this book. Nonetheless, it would be remiss of us not to inform readers that occasionally a patient will have a planned outpatient procedure that turns out to require hospitalization. This may occur for several reasons, on the continuum from mild to severe. At the very mild end of the spectrum: an *ambulatory* outpatient surgery was planned for midafternoon, but the start was delayed to an evening procedure and the allocated observation time period ran out. Thus hospital staff and resources were required to "finish" the observation by keeping the patient overnight. Sometimes operations have complications, and patients need more services than a surgicenter can offer or need to be observed for longer than is possible in a surgicenter. The most common reason for admission overnight is that pain cannot be controlled with oral medication. Sometimes a patient is sicker than originally realized, or a new ailment is discovered requiring emergency care. If you have a scheduled outpatient operation, it is prudent to ask your surgeon about the contingency plan if you require admission.

CHAPTER 14

Unplanned Surgery

Many people will leave the hospital having had a surgery they did not plan for. You might come in to the emergency room for abdominal pain and be found to have a small hole in your bowel, which could lead to having a part of the bowel surgically removed. You might come in for dizziness and be found to have a slow heart rate that requires insertion of a pacemaker. You might come in for chest pain and end up needing coronary bypass to restore blood flow to the vessels nourishing the heart. The emergency room team's job is to figure out which specialty needs to be consulted to see if your situation requires admission. Sometimes there is an immediate need for an operation, and the surgical team will be alerted. However, often the source of the problem is not immediately clear. It may take many tests and several consultations to determine whether surgery is warranted.

MEDICAL CLEARANCE

Unplanned surgery can be *emergent* (indicating an emergency) or *semi-emergent* (urgent). Unlike with planned surgery, there is less time to medically *optimize* (prepare to obtain the best result) the patient prior to the surgery. In a true emergency situation, there is no time for medical optimization and no requirement for medical clearance since usually the patient is in imminent risk of death without the surgery. In a semi-urgent situation, there is a little more time to properly risk-stratify the patient. *Risk stratification* is a process performed by the medical attending physician or cardiologist. The doctor will look at your underlying medical conditions and your ability to exercise without symptoms, and determine if there is a need for further workup before proceeding to surgery. Common tests ordered include echocardiograms, stress tests, and cardiac catheterizations.

TYPICAL UNPLANNED SURGERIES

Following are some of the most common unplanned surgeries:

1. Bowel perforation (small hole) repair from either *diverticulitis* (inflammation of small pouches in the colon—large intestine) or *colitis* (inflammation in the colon).
2. Cardiac bypass—you come in with chest pain and end up with an angiogram that indicates you have many blocked vessels in your heart. Blockages that cannot be addressed with angioplasty and stents will require *coronary bypass surgery.*
3. Any type of trauma, which includes falls leading to broken hips and legs in the elderly.
4. *Video-assisted thorascopic surgery (VATS)*—surgery to get into the lungs with a small

Medical Clearance for Surgery

There is always the possibility that you may need to have surgery while you are in the hospital. If this is the case, you will need to be cleared for it. Most of the time, this clearance can be done by the attending medical physician. The attending will ask you multiple questions about your exercise tolerance, history of heart and lung disease, and prior surgeries. The attending will also review your blood work and your electrocardiogram. On the basis of these results, the attending may ask for further testing, such as an echocardiogram or stress test (described in chapter 8). It is also possible that the medical attending may ask for a cardiologist to evaluate you to make recommendations. Prior to surgery, you will also be evaluated by the anesthesiologist, since undergoing anesthesia is typically one of the riskier aspects of the operation. The doctors, nurses, NPs, and PAs, through all the questioning and additional testing, want to make sure that you have the best chance for a good outcome with surgery.

camera to perform necessary biopsies and surgical procedures. This is often done in patients with lung cancer and complicated pneumonia.

5. Valve replacement—shortness of breath and chest pain may result if one of the valves in your heart is not working correctly, and the valve needs to be fixed or replaced.
6. Gallbladder or appendix removal.

BEFORE UNPLANNED SURGERY

Consent for Surgery

Consent for surgery will be obtained from you if you are in a condition (conscious, alert, and oriented) to sign. If you are unable to sign, the consent can be signed by the next of kin—your spouse, adult child, or parent. If the surgery is emergent and lifesaving, consent does not need to be obtained. This is common for trauma cases such as a serious car or motorcycle accident. If you are able to sign your own consent, the surgeon will explain the risks, benefits, and alternatives to the surgery. There is a separate consent process for anesthesia. The anesthesiologist will explain procedures and risks and will obtain consent from the patient if possible or next of kin if the patient cannot sign. The anesthesiologist can also forgo requiring consent to provide lifesaving procedures in the event of the need for immediate surgery. For extremely time-sensitive emergencies, the anesthesiologist will begin his or her work in the ER; protecting the airway is the primary consideration. The *endotracheal tube* (tube into the airway) can be placed in the ER prior to transporting the patient to the operating room.

From the Emergency Department (Emergency Room) to the Operating Room

It is possible to end up in the OR from many different starting places in the hospital. Emergency surgeries often come straight from the emergency department (ED), also called the emergency room (ER). For example, patients who come in with trauma will be evaluated in the ER by the surgical team and often be taken straight to the OR. In the event of several trauma cases coming in together, a "code trauma" will be called over the hospital intercom. When this occurs, it will alert surgeons, nurses, and anesthesiologists to report to the ER immediately, bypassing the usual phone calls back and forth to bring the team in for consultations. This is considered an all-out emergency. Many other conditions requiring surgical intervention will require consultation with surgeons. In a teaching hospital, the first contact will be with a resident, who will report the findings of his or her physical examination, combined with a report of the patient's history, to the attending surgeon. The need for emergency surgery occurs in a very confusing and rushed atmosphere. Do not be afraid to speak up and ask what is going on.

From the Cardiac Catheterization Lab to the OR

Sometimes a procedure to investigate one condition leads to another. For example, you might have an *angiogram* (an X-ray of the blood vessels) for chest pain. If the angiogram finds that you have the three vessels feeding your heart blocked, you may need a coronary bypass. This is an open heart surgery for which you will be admitted. If you need to go the OR right away, other cases will get bumped. If your surgery is not urgent, your surgeon needs to book an OR time. Sometimes this can take a few days.

Getting on the Surgeon's Schedule

The creation of a surgeon's schedule is a complex process managed by surgical schedulers. This scheduler may not have any formal medical training but is required to juggle the surgeon's OR schedule times by taking into account planned surgeries, emergency surgeries, semi-emergency surgeries, patient medical clearance, availability of the operating room, and sometimes the availability of the surgeon's physician assistant if that is the practice of the surgeon. The scheduler may also have to coordinate with presurgical testing staff, insurance precertification, and the anesthesiology office. Certain surgical specialties are geared toward incorporating emergency cases into the schedule. Cardiothoracic and trauma surgeons will frequently bump planned surgeries to accommodate a patient's operation that cannot wait if the patient's condition is life-threatening. For patients admitted with a semi-emergent need for surgery, every effort will be made to fit the patient into the schedule as expeditiously as possible. This is both for the safety of the patient and to contain the cost of extra "bed days" while the patient is waiting around for surgery.

The Wait

Millie's son was concerned about her sudden shortness of breath. Mom was in her eighties and on blood pressure and cholesterol medication. Although she did not want to go to the ER on a bright and beautiful spring day, her son insisted. The nurse at the ER did a quick exam and alerted the emergency medicine doctor, who requested an EKG to look at Millie's heart rhythm and ordered blood tests to see if Millie had had a heart attack. Before long, Millie was in the cardiac catheterization lab to get an angiogram, a procedure by an interventional cardiologist to visualize the heart and vessels. It soon became apparent from the EKG, the angiogram, and the blood tests, that Millie had had a mild heart attack and that she would require surgery to allow better blood flow to the heart. When would this happen? Millie was eager to get the surgery over and done with, but she was told it would be at least a day or so. She found herself in the coronary care unit on a heart monitor. Millie's case was urgent but not an outright emergency. The cardiothoracic surgeon would make room for her on the schedule but not immediately.

NPO before Surgery

This is a Latin phrase: *non per os* meaning nothing by mouth. If you are scheduled for a surgery there will be no eating or drinking (*NPO*) for at least six hours before the operation. If you vomit with food in the stomach while under anesthesia, you run the risk of getting *aspiration* pneumonia. Usually patients are allowed to take their daily medications with a sip of water. **It is extremely important that if you are told not to take any food or drink, you comply with this.** Ask your doctor to clarify which medications are approved before surgery and which must be avoided. What happens when the surgery is an emergency? The NPO rule goes out the door, since the risk of aspiration is outweighed by the benefit of getting the patient under anesthesia and beginning the operation as quickly as possible. This process if called *rapid sequence induction*; the anesthesiologist will follow strict protocols to minimize the risk of complications.

Antibiotics

For many types of surgery, you will be given an antibiotic before surgery to prevent infection because surgery can put you at risk for infections. The doses, types, and duration of the antibiotic medication vary for the type of operation and your medical status prior to surgery.

SERVICE CHANGES: WHO'S IN CHARGE?

Understanding who the team is and who is in charge of your care during a hospital stay can be quite confusing. This is especially true in teaching hospitals, where there are personnel in multiple stages of training involved in patient care. Often patients are on the *medicine service* (the general name for primary care and specialties concerned with internal medicine that will be responsible for rendering care) and will end up going for a surgery. If it is an uncomplicated surgery (for example, gall bladder removal, repair of a simple bone fracture) and you have other medical conditions such as diabetes or kidney disease, you will usually go back to the medicine service. In practical terms, this means that even if you have had an operation, an internist has responsibility for your care after the surgery is completed. If it is a complicated surgery requiring close follow-up by the surgeon (for example, removal of part of the colon), you will remain on the surgical service, where a surgeon has responsibility for your overall care. The surgeon may ask for a medicine consult to help manage any existing medical issues. The more complicated the patient issues are, the more likely that multiple consults will be called and that several specialists will be involved. It is possible that you will move through different services during an inpatient stay. It may not always be evident which specialty or service has ultimate responsibility for care. If your medical team has not been forthcoming with this information, we encourage you to ask your health care team members who is in charge and to explain the various consultants' roles. Determining the responsible provider for your care is a key step to help you advocate for the best possible care during your stay. Learning this fact will save time if you have questions or if problems arise. For a more detailed explanation, please turn to the first section of chapter 6.

YOUR ROOM

If you have been admitted through the emergency room and sent directly to the operating room, you will get to your room after surgery. If you have had a semi-emergent surgery, you may have spent a day or two in a room while waiting for surgery. Unfortunately, during very high-demand times in the hospital, some patients will get stuck in an ER bed while waiting for surgery—we hope this does not happen to you. It is very likely that you will not return to your original room and bed for several reasons: allocating beds in the hospital is another one of those complex processes and is subject to many factors. If you will be in the OR and PACU for many hours and your bed is needed for another patient, it will be given away. Another possible scenario is that you have been admitted to one type of service—for example, medicine, neurology, interventional cardiology (cardiac catheterization lab)—but after the need for surgery is determined, you are placed on the surgical service and will go to a surgery unit and bed. As always, the larger and more complex the hospital, the more specialized units there will be. Surgical nursing care is different from medical or neurological nursing care, so when there is an opportunity to group similar types of patients together in one location, efficiency and care are improved, and you will benefit from this expertise. However, all the possible room changes may be disorienting. If you have found yourself close to the window or in a private space in your first room and you end up in a four-bed room near the door, closer to hallway noise, you may not be completely happy. It is perfectly reasonable to inquire where you will go after surgery and to request your preferences. We cannot guarantee that requests will be honored, but it never hurts to try.

AFTER SURGERY

Post-anesthesia Care Unit (PACU, Recovery Room)

The *post-anesthesia care unit (PACU)* is where you go right after surgery while you are still waking up from the anesthesia. Anesthesiologists supervise care for you in this unit. The nurses, doctors, and nurse anesthetists need to make sure that you successfully come out of anesthesia and are able to breathe on your own. This is usually where family members are first allowed to lay eyes on you after surgery at the discretion of the care team once you are stabilized. Although you may be drowsy or nauseated and may not remember much about receiving brief visits, it is usually very comforting for families and friends to spend a moment with you or to stay and hold your hand before you are transferred to another unit. On occasion, following certain surgical procedures, you might be brought directly from the OR to the ICU by the anesthesiologist. Recovery location may also depend on how many spaces and nurses are available in the PACU and also on the time of day that you are emerging from surgery. When operations take place in the middle of the night, the PACU may not be adequately staffed to manage patients coming out of surgery. In this case, recovery from anesthesia may occur on the surgical unit or ICU but under the supervision of trained staff.

Contact with the Surgical Team after Surgery

At least once a day, someone from the surgical team will *round* (come to see you) to check the *dressing* and *drains* and will make sure that the *surgical wound* (where the incision was made) is healing well. In addition to these rounds, the nurse will contact the surgeon if there are any concerns about the wound or your general recovery. Many recovery processes after surgery occur by predetermined protocols—as soon as the patient achieves a certain milestone, the next step in the process can occur. For example, on the first postoperative day, you will be encouraged to stand up and shuffle to a chair. This will set you up for a short walk around your room later that day or the following day. In a similar fashion, your diet and pain control will also move through stages as you progress toward normalcy.

Pain Control

Patients who have undergone an operation will typically experience pain afterward. As you can imagine—particularly with "open" procedures in which incisions are made through skin, muscle, and bone—your pain can be quite severe. Many factors influence patients' experience of pain. Males and females display tolerance differently, personality plays a key role, and even ethnicity and culture influence pain tolerance. Huge advances in anesthetic techniques and medications have changed the experience of pain after surgery.

Pain Medications

If you listen to the news or read the newspaper, you will know that opioid overuse and abuse has become an epic problem in the United States. Therefore, there is an increasing effort to find nonnarcotic approaches to dealing with pain. Many research studies are currently being conducted to discover "opioid- sparing" methods to reduce pain. Different types and locations of anesthesia are being tested. Giving nonnarcotic medications such as NSAIDs (ibuprofen and naproxen sodium) and acetaminophen during the surgery is also being tested, with the idea to prevent the onset of pain and to block the pain receptors before the pain begins. Depending on the type of surgery, the anesthesiologist may administer a nerve block in the operating room to control your pain and to prevent the need for pain medication.

Patient-Controlled Analgesia (PCA)

After surgery, many patients will be able to "order" their own pain medication through a *PCA*, which is a ***patient-controlled analgesia*** pump that delivers pain medication, usually a narcotic, to your blood through your IV when you push a button. To prevent overdose, timing and dosage limits are preset. Sometimes, patients experience extreme pain to the point where they are extremely uncomfortable even when the PCA is delivering medication. If you are really miserable, it is important to let the nurse and other health care professionals know about it. Everyone has different pain medication needs and requires different doses of pain medication. It is important to make the hospital staff aware that you are in pain so they can adjust the dose or even change the medication.

Anticoagulant Medications

If there is time prior to an unplanned surgery, *anticoagulants* (blood thinners) will be discontinued. However, if the patient is in imminent danger, surgeons will operate regardless of the patient's anticoagulation status since the risk of delaying surgery outweighs the risk of bleeding. There are certain surgical procedures that put patients at very high risk for developing blood clots; these include hip-fracture repair, as well as cardiac and abdominal surgery. Therefore, soon after surgery, and if bleeding has slowed down or stopped, it is likely that you will either be put back on a blood thinner or aspirin or be started on one of these medications to prevent *venous thromboembolism* (blood clot). A clot results when the blood is not flowing well. Often clots form in the legs, where people may or may not experience symptoms (pain, swelling, redness, tenderness). This is called a *deep vein thrombosis*, or *DVT*. The real danger exists when a clot travels from your legs or your arms to your lungs. This is called a *pulmonary embolism (PE)*. If this occurs, you may experience pain in your chest or difficulty breathing. Very rarely it can cause sudden death. After surgery you will be prescribed injections or pills of anticoagulant medication. You may also be put on *sequential compression devices (Venodynes),* either with or without anticoagulant medication. While you are in bed, these devices surround your leg and periodically compress them to keep the blood flowing well. There are also *TEDS (compression stockings)* that you can wear when you're not in bed. If you are able to walk, and if your doctors and nurses encourage you to do so, you should take frequent and vigorous walks, which will also help to reduce the risk of clots, since immobilization increases the chance of developing a DVT.

Diet after Surgery

Depending on the type of surgery and what organs and body parts are affected, food will be gradually reintroduced after your surgery. If there has been a very major operation, particularly if any of the digestive organs have been operated on, the reintroduction may be very gradual. Often after surgery involving the bowels, the doctors and nurses will check you daily to see whether you are making bowel sounds again and passing gas. These signs indicate that the bowel is functioning again and ready for the reintroduction of food. During this time, the doctors and nurses will evaluate whether your digestive tract is ready for more of a challenge. You might start with clear liquids and ices and then move to solid foods as the staff determines that your digestive tract is working normally. It could be several days until you are ready for a normal diet. A major complication after surgery is *postoperative ileus*. This is a condition in which the bowel slows down so much that it is as if there is a mechanical obstruction (blockage). When this occurs, your belly will become severely distended; you can become nauseated and vomit. If there is a postoperative ileus, there may be a need to place an *NG* tube for decompression. As in all things, any questions should be directed to your nurse or your health care provider.

TIP   Visitors

If you have come into the hospital without planning for surgery, you may not have had time to reflect on your feelings about receiving visitors. Furthermore, if you are in the hospital for an unexpected operation, you will not have had time to educate family and friends about what you are permitted to do or eat postoperatively. Your job is to recover, and undue stress may impede recovery. It will be important to have a family member or friend close by to bring comfort, help you, and advocate for you. Please encourage visits (if not overnight stays) from the individuals who you think will best fulfill those roles. Remember that it is not your job to entertain visitors or assure them that you will be fine. Having nonessential visitors initially may feel intrusive. Take care of yourself first. Visits can take place later, or at home. Visitors may mean well but can be distressing, noisy, and nosy.

Discharge after Unplanned Surgery

If you have come into the hospital without plans for surgery, you will not have thought about what will happen after discharge or have had time to research rehab facilities. Often patients who have undergone surgery are not quite ready to return to the home environment immediately follow-ing a hospital stay; these patients may require a transitional period for recuperation in a subacute facility where they will be monitored and will receive therapies. The question of whether you will be sent to a rehabili-tation facility (also called subacute facility or a skilled nursing facility) is dependent on many factors and is part of a changing medical landscape due to insurance and government payers (Medicare and Medicaid), reg-ulations, and compensation. In addition, there are regional differences in where patients go after the hospital. In short, we are unable to predict or generalize whether you will return to your previous living arrangement directly after the hospital stay since there are so many factors involved. For surgery patients, the discharge disposition considerations include the physical layout of your home environment (such as stairs), whether your muscles have to be retrained by experts (physical and occupational therapy), and your baseline health status. Generally, and as we would ex-pect, a younger, previously healthy person will need fewer services after discharge, and an older, sicker patient will need more. Finding out the best possible match between the patient and the rehab center is the job of the case managers. We discuss many more details about discharge plan-ning and suitability of discharge to home rather than a rehab facility in chapter 15.

TIP   Participating in the Search for the Right Rehab Center

It is important that you and your family members participate in the iden-tification and location of the facility to which you will be discharged if you are not returning home. Ideally the facility should be close to where your family and friends can visit regularly. If you or a family member has had an unplanned surgery, it may be helpful to ask friends and neighbors about their experiences in local rehab centers since there can be a great deal of variability in services offered and atmosphere among facilities. The case managers will be helpful, but ultimately a visit to look around the rehab will be instructive.

CHAPTER 15

Discharge

Believe it or not, you are being evaluated for discharge just as soon as you enter the hospital. This is the area of specialization for *case managers*, usually nurses, who might work with social workers and confer with doctors, nurse practitioners, physician assistants, and therapists about what kind of care will be required after your inpatient stay. Case managers (*discharge planners*) work closely with the facilities to which you may be transferred.

On the basis of information gleaned from the medical charts, discussions with the care team, and previous experience with similar conditions, these trained case managers put together a good big picture of what you need after you are discharged from the hospital. They have links and relationships with other care settings and all kinds of health care professionals. Just as soon as you are admitted, the case manager knows about you and is on the case. The reason for this early attention is to pave the way for a smooth transition after your hospital stay.

Increasingly, medically hospitalized patients are older and sicker and have shorter lengths of stay in the hospital. Elective surgical patients are a different group entirely and have different needs after discharge. However, just because someone has a short stay in the hospital does not mean that he or she is completely ready to go home. A fairly recent development in health care is for patients to leave the hospital to go to a less acute care setting. Often this is a rehabilitation (rehab)center.

For older or disabled patients, a *skilled nursing facility (SNF)* might be called for. The goal is to ensure that patients have a smooth recovery and do not need to be readmitted for a relapse or reinjury. Although the hospital is just the right place for very sick patients or patients requiring surgery, it is the wrong place to linger when recuperating. There are many reasons for this. The hospital environment harbors many germs, and the longer your stay, the more likely you are to become infected; the expense of being in the hospital (assumed mostly by insurance carriers and the government) is enormous; and as discussed in chapter 1, there is a possibility that patients, particularly those in a weakened state, could fall victim to a medical error.

If you are well enough to leave the hospital and can get adequate care in the home or other setting, usually the best situation will be for you to get in and out of the hospital as quickly as is safe and feasible. In the current era of enormous financial health care burden, there is pressure on hospitals and health care professionals to move patients through the inpatient stay quite rapidly. In fact, in the early 1980s, Medicare implemented a classification system called diagnostic-related groups (DRGs) that provides hospitals with information about expected lengths of stay for various illnesses and related conditions. This information, in turn, provides "guidance" about how much reimbursement the hospital gets. As a consequence, patients may at times be rushed out of the hospital earlier than would be optimal. This topic is an area of debate and controversy, not surprisingly.

ACTIVITIES OF DAILY LIVING (ADLs)

One of the reasons you may need to go to a rehabilitation facility is that you cannot accomplish your *activities of daily living (ADLs)* without assistance. These activities define what makes you independent. Can you dress, feed, and toilet yourself? These are key indicators of your functional ability. If you cannot do these things, you are dependent on someone else, such as a full time live-in aide or family member. Or you may need to live in a skilled nursing facility.

THE PROCESS OF DISCHARGE PLANNING

The discharge planning process takes into account several factors: your baseline status, which means how you were before the hospital stay; how well you manage daily activities alone or with help; whether family and other caregivers (such as paid aides) are available to see to your needs after the hospital; resources for medication and nutrition; and transportation home. Some patients will need some services after going home, such as a visiting nurse, nurse's aide, or physical therapy. Patients who go home on IV antibiotics or need injections after the hospital stay will require special attention from nurses.

There are many variables that enter into the decision about where you are placed after the hospital: your ADL status, the availability of a rehab or nursing home bed, support from family and friends, the distance from your home to outpatient services, and the amount the insurance company is willing to reimburse or pay for services and for how long.

REHABILITATION

Patients who have been confined to a bed for many days will experience deconditioning of the muscles. They might need to practice standing and walking again before they are steady enough on their feet to go home safely. They may not be able to feed or dress themselves until they have regained sufficient strength. Deconditioning happens in other organs of the body as well. After a heart attack or pneumonia, it may take more effort to breathe; therefore, patients will need to slowly reintroduce themselves to exertion. Often, trained therapists will be necessary to help this process along.

For surgery patients, the discharge disposition considerations include the physical layout of the home environment (such as stairs), whether muscles have to be retrained by experts (physical and occupational therapy), and the baseline health status of the patient. Generally, and as we would expect, a younger, previously healthy person will need fewer services after discharge than an older, sicker patient. Stroke patients who have suffered loss of movement, in particular, tend to need more rehabilitation services after discharge—most often speech, physical therapy, and occupational therapy. Finding out the best possible match for you and any rehab center that may be required is the job of the case managers. These trained professionals might begin making phone calls to facilities the moment you arrive at the hospital.

TIP   Clothes

You need clothes when at a rehab facility. Most people, however, when admitted to the hospital end up without their street clothes. This is because family members are often told to take home all your valuables, so usually your clothes end up going home too. Ask a family member to bring your clothes and a pair of comfortable shoes for the day you are going to the rehab facility. If it is during the winter, ask for your coat, hat, and gloves. If you do not have these things, you will end up being transferred in a hospital gown wrapped in a blanket!

TIP   Finding the Right Rehab Facility for the Patient

The case managers will work diligently to get the patient placement in rehab. They will match up the needs of the patient and the availability of a bed (which means a spot in the facility). There is a great amount of variability in rehab centers, and if at all possible, it is optimal for family members to actually visit several places where the patient might stay, particularly if it will be for more than a few days. If you are planning on visiting a family member in a rehab facility, you will have to consider how you will get there, how far it is from home, and how friendly and receptive the facility is to visitors. To make the best decision, these factors should be combined with observations about reputation, cleanliness, and frequency of therapies. We recognize that "interviewing" rehab facilities can be stressful but urge you to make an in-person visit nonetheless.

SKILLED NURSING FACILITIES

Skilled nursing facilities often play the dual role of both nursing home and rehab facility. In practical terms, this means that long-term elderly patients who live at the facility usually remain until the end of their lives. In these facilities there may also be a true rehabilitation section with short-stay beds for patients who need therapies and services after hospitalization prior to returning home. Sometimes a family may recognize that it is time to start transitioning their loved one into a long-term skilled nursing facility. As this process can be complicated both from a financial and a legal standpoint, patients are often sent to the rehab portion of the facility and are eventually moved into the long-term care area.

> **TIP**   Determining the Best Rehab or Skilled Nursing Facility for Long-Term Care Placement
>
> The decision to transition a family member to a long-term care facility may be stressful, difficult, and sad. At best it is complex and requires careful consultation and planning. Guidance should be sought from multiple sources: health care providers, social workers, and discharge planners. It may also be useful to discuss the experiences of friends and family members who have gone through this process and to get their recommendations. For financial considerations, Medicare and the insurance company will furnish information about coverage. It will also be important to explore the ratio of nurses and nursing assistants to patients, as many facilities are not adequately staffed. An Internet search using the term "finding the right long-term care facility" may provide insights, but you should ignore sponsored sites and instead concentrate on consumer-oriented sites, which should be less subject to advertising bias.

What Rebab Center Is Best?

Michael's elderly father had suffered a debilitating stroke. Now his dad would need significant rehab services to regain function. They were fortunate to live in a city with many opportunities for fine care. But how to choose the right one? The case managers suggested two rehab centers. One had a national reputation but was very far from Mike's home. Mike did not know how he could see his father every day. The other facility was almost but not quite as well regarded, but it was close to Mike's home, so he knew he could visit Dad every day without fail. As Mike soon discovered, there is no one right answer. As in all things, compromises and trade-offs would have to be made. Mike decided to ask the doctors and nurses and social worker to help with this difficult decision; this was a good way to alleviate any guilt he might feel if he chose the more distant center, where he might not visit as often as he wished.

CONNECTING WITH YOUR DOCTOR OR OTHER HEALTH CARE PROVIDERS AFTER DISCHARGE

It is vital to your recuperation to have good communication with your doctor or other health care provider after you leave the hospital. He or she may not be aware that you have been in the hospital, let alone know the reason why. A follow-up visit is in order. Sometimes this process will be initiated by the hospital staff, but more often than not, it is incumbent on you to set up a follow-up visit shortly after hospital discharge to ensure that all is going according to plan for your recovery.

MEDICATION (AGAIN!!!!)

It is very possible that after a hospital stay, your medication list and dosages— for example, antibiotics or short-term *anticoagulation* (blood-thinning) medications—will have changed, maybe temporarily but also likely for a longer duration. Getting used to new medications, new doses, and new schedules may be confusing and overwhelming. Furthermore, there may be not only changes but substitutions in your medications during the hospital stay. For this reason, it is important that you become aware of which medications are duplications or redundant so that you are not doubling up on certain ones. On the other hand, the doctors at the hospital may have stopped medications that interfere with treatment or procedures. You will need to restart these after returning home. It will take some extra organization and effort on your part, including filling prescriptions, reading new instructions for taking these medications, and setting up a pill minder. Generally, before you leave the hospital, a nurse will go over your list of medications with you and a family member in the medication reconciliation process. You will have this in writing.

TIP   Helping Elderly Patients Sort Out Medication after Discharge

It is not uncommon for elderly people to become confused about medication, and this confusion can be exacerbated by a hospital stay. Medications may be added, changed, discontinued, and substituted, and doses may be adjusted. For caregivers of these patients, it is crucial to get involved during the hospital stay to prevent problems after discharge. It will be helpful to have a list of prehospital medications to compare with the medications on discharge. Some elderly patients who were competent to self-administer medications before their hospital admission will be temporarily—if not permanently—unable to continue to manage on their own after a hospital stay. It will be important to determine early whether this will be an issue in order to involve visiting nurses or other help in the home. If questions arise about medication redundancy or unusual side effects, the health care team is equipped to provide answers. Do not hesitate to pose questions in the hospital and the rehab or skilled nursing facility. For patients returning home, the local pharmacist can be an important resource about medication questions.

GOALS OF CARE

There are multiple points in a hospital stay at which it is appropriate to discuss the goals of care for the patient. Of course it is optimal to have these conversations with your loved ones before a hospital stay even occurs. One should make every effort to designate a *health care proxy* (a person who will make medical decisions if you cannot make them for yourself) and draft a *living will* (a document stating what you do and do not want for yourself—e.g., resuscitation, tube feeding). Unfortunately, most people have not done this, and therefore these decisions are often forced on family members at the time of highest emotional distress. If you or your family member is critically ill, you should expect doctors and other health care professionals to question you about your wishes for resuscitation. They want to know whether you want to be shocked if your heart should stop, and whether you want to be placed on a ventilator if you stop breathing. Typically a nurse will initiate this conversation about a *do not resuscitate*

(*DNR*) order and will provide written material to give you some time to reflect. Believe it or not, many patients answer no to these questions. Many people feel they have already lived a good life and do not want to end up attached to machines. No doctor can guarantee that once a patient is placed on these machines, the doctors and nurses will be able to wean him or her off them. Most large medical centers now have *palliative care* teams. These are generally made up of a palliative care physician, nurse practitioners or physician assistants, nurses, social workers, and chaplains. The palliative care teams are excellent at family meetings and helping to bring family members together to help make these important decisions. (This topic is discussed in greater detail in the section on end-of-life care in chapter 12.)

MONITORING FOR WARNING SIGNS AND SYMPTOMS WHEN YOU ARE HOME

Depending on the reason for your hospital stay, you may have to monitor your medical condition when you go home. As part of the discharge process, you will be told what signs and symptoms to watch out for when at home. If you notice one of them, you should be prompted to call your doctor. For example, if you were admitted to the hospital for a heart attack, you may be advised to call if you have chest pain or shortness of breath. If you were admitted with a urinary tract infection, you might be on the alert for burning when you urinate. If you do not understand the instructions given on discharge, do not be afraid to speak up and say so. As always, it is important to have another set of ears to help integrate important medical information. In addition, even if you are given written instructions about what warning signs to look for, writing things down can help reinforce the message.

TIP   Warning Signs and Symptoms after Discharge

Warning signs and symptoms will be on a continuum of urgency. Some symptoms will warrant a call to 911, while others can wait a couple of days to see if they are part of the normal recovery process. Before discharge, clarify with your providers which signs and symptoms are part of the normal recovery process and which may signal an impending emergency. When in doubt, call your health care provider.

CHAPTER 16

Some Final Thoughts

SHOWING APPRECIATION FOR THE HEALTH CARE TEAM, LETTERS, GIFTS OF FOOD

Unlike some other fields, health care is an around-the-clock endeavor. Health care providers must work shifts through days and nights, holidays and weekends because illness and injury do not care about time. The health care team gives up precious moments with their loved ones to care for yours. Even when the system does not work as well as it could, it is important to recognize the individuals working within the system who are doing their best day in and day out. There are many ways to show appreciation for the team taking care of you. In our opinion, the most important is really just a simple thank you. Thank yous can go such a long way when people are stressed and working hard. Thank you notes or letters are also greatly appreciated. A letter of praise for an individual who has gone above and beyond will go in the personnel file. Gifts of food are almost always appreciated by the floor staff. Others gifts are not necessary, and in fact, most medical institutions have policies about what kinds of gifts can be accepted. Do not feel insulted if a gift you offer is turned down and the recipient suggests that if you are happy with your care, you could instead consider writing a letter to the hospital administrators or making a donation to the institution.

TIP   Gifts of Food

The way to anyone's heart is through the stomach. For people who work long hours taking care of patients, a food treat is a welcome break. When we have loved ones in the hospital, we always bring a food item to show our appreciation. The gift you bring does not have to be fancy; a commercially prepared box of donut holes says "thanks." We have seen this simple gift but also have seen elaborate deli spreads delivered for the entire unit. Here are few pointers:

- Include a well-marked card or simply write on the box to indicate who the gift is from. You would say something like "from the family of John Doe in room 555 with our appreciation."
- Do not wait until discharge to bring your food gift. You want to show appreciation DURING the stay.
- If your family member will be on the unit for more than a couple of days (and consequently will be cared for by different staff from many shifts), it is better to bring something simple each day or every couple of days. You might bring boxes of chocolates.
- Avoid home-prepared gifts of food. It is more thoughtful to bring in something from a known store, bakery, or restaurant so the recipients do not have to be concerned about the source.
- Drop off the food and note at the nursing station with the unit clerks. They know what to do!

Bringing in Food for the Staff

When my mother was admitted to the ICU for a pulmonary embolus and bilateral arterial clots in the legs, it was a touch-and-go situation, and we did not believe she would pull through. To make matters worse, her body rejected the blood transfusion. She was in pain, the family was terrified, and even the doctors and nurses were baffled about how the clots had traveled through the filter. (It turned out that there was a previously undetected hole in her heart.) Well, Mom is tough, the vascular surgeons were superb, and intensivists premedicated her with Benadryl so that her body would accept the transfusion. The nurses, respiratory therapists, and other professionals and health care staff taking care of her were also amazing. She got better. During her ICU stay, we wanted to let the staff know how grateful we were for their knowledge, skill, the attention and care they had given her, and the comfort they provided to us. We asked the unit clerk where the staff liked to order their pizza from, and at lunchtime, we called in an order for a few boxes. For the rest of the day, nurses, PAs, and other floor staff stopped into the room to thank us; even the staff not taking care of Mom now knew who this patient was. We got to tell our story over and over, with the knowledge that the health care team would keep a special eye on this patient.—*Sara Merwin*

USING THE INTERNET TO GET INFORMATION ABOUT ILLNESSES

With the advent of the Internet, patients and the rest of society have the world of knowledge at their fingertips. This can be both beneficial and harmful. If you are computer savvy, it is hard not to be tempted to look up your disease and information about your current situation. There is a lot of information on the web but also a tremendous amount of misinformation and misleading information. Medical professionals, as part of their training, are instructed on how to properly search the available literature for the most evidence-based information and how to properly interpret that information. If you have chosen to get information from the web, please be sure to discuss it with your physician and other providers. They can help verify the validity of your sources and help you interpret the findings.

PRIVATE-DUTY NURSES

Nursing ratios vary from unit to unit and from hospital to hospital. Some patients may require more attention than can always be provided to them. This is especially true of elderly patients with dementia, who can often become agitated in the hospital. They may need to be redirected often and require help with basic necessities such as bathing and feeding. Hiring private-duty nurses is a way to provide extra care during the hospital stay. These nurses are hired through a private agency and are paid for out of pocket by the family. Unfortunately, they can be expensive. If you are interested in hiring a private-duty nurse, the hospital may have a list of agencies that have previously provided services. A private-duty nurse can function only according to the rules of each hospital. For example, many hospitals will allow only the actual hospital-employed nurse to dispense the patient's medications.

Someone with the skills of a nurse is not always needed. Companions are an excellent choice, and a less expensive option, to help with elderly patients. They can keep patients company, reorient them when needed, and help with meals, grooming, and hygiene. A companion can also alert the nurse if extra attention by the health care team is required.

MEDICAL FRIENDS AND FAMILY AS RESOURCES

It is reasonable to be concerned about family members or ourselves during a hospital stay. This may be because medical errors are a major concern or because most people are out of their comfort zone in a medical milieu. Some of us have friends or family members who work in health care, either as doctors, nurses, physician assistants, or other health care professionals. It is normal for us to turn to them for advice or help, particularly if we are being taken care of at their institution. However, accepting advice from providers not actually caring for you can have an upside and a downside. The upside is that there is often an extra pair of eyes watching and trying to make sure nothing goes wrong. The downside is that this extra pair of eyes is biased, and this can lead health care teams to make biased medical decisions instead of decisions grounded in evidence. In addition, patients may be caught in the middle of conflicting advice about care.

HOW YOU CAN DEAL WITH A MEDICAL ERROR

In the first chapter we discussed medical errors and the epidemic of patients suffering the consequences—often fatal—from these mistakes.

Errors of commission are ones in which something specifically incorrect was done or given to a patient. An *error of omission*, on the other hand, means that the patient did not get the medication or procedure or provision of care necessary, or that something varied from what the medical profession calls the *standard of care*. What if you believe that you or a loved one has sustained a medical error during a hospital stay? Here are our recommendations for the appropriate course of action:

> Address your concern right away with the person in charge of your care.
> Ask him or her to explain why the error occurred and the possible consequences.
> Ask what will be done now to protect you and to correct the error.
> Ask what steps the providers are taking after this error to ensure your health remains intact.
> Ask what the providers will do to ensure the same mistake does not happen again to you or another patient.
> Expect an apology from the individual or team members responsible for the medical error.

If you are not satisfied with the answers you receive, escalate your complaints to the administration of the hospital. It will be important to follow up with a letter stating the complaint so that you have a record. Hospitals have risk management departments to deal with medical errors; in many states there are requirements to report errors. There are also many governmental and private organizations currently collecting information on medical errors and proving guidance to patients who have sustained an error. Of course, depending on the severity of the error and the result, you may need to contact a lawyer to pursue a claim.

PARTICIPATE IN YOUR CARE!

Speaking Up

During the writing of this book, I had occasion to take my own advice. There was a medical problem requiring a visit to my primary care physician, an internist. The doctor examined me and took a recent history to give her clues about what might be causing my symptoms. Not surprisingly, it turned out the diagnosis wasn't immediately evident and I would need further tests; the doctor suggested a CT scan. As it turns out, I had had quite a few diagnostic tests involving radiation exposure this year and had been advised by a radiologist to seek other imaging methods. So I told the doctor I did not want to have a CT scan and cited the reasons why. Between the two of us, we worked out another solution—mutually satisfactory. She wasn't affronted, and I had done my job to both protect myself and make my wishes clear. To be fair, I had chosen this doctor precisely because I sought a partnership (as opposed to a dictatorship). Nonetheless, we are all entitled to obtain the best possible health care from our providers by asking questions and speaking up for ourselves.—*Sara Merwin*

We hope that you learned something from this book and that you will find it a useful resource when you or a loved one is hospitalized. We will leave you with the following message, which is so central to our philosophy about how, in the modern era, patients must accept responsibility for their own care: when it comes to choosing treatment options and making decisions about medical care, it is vitally important for you to express your own wishes and to be a full participant.

GLOSSARY

abdominal ultrasound. Imaging method using radio waves to look at the liver, the ducts that run through it, gallbladder, spleen, kidneys, and bladder.

ablate. To remove or destroy the tissue that is causing a problem.

ACTH. A substance found in the pituitary gland that controls steroid production by the adrenal glands.

ACTH stimulation test. A test that evaluates pituitary and adrenal gland function by measuring a hormone produced by the adrenal gland.

activities of daily living (ADLs). Activities that define a person's independence, such as feeding, toileting, and household tasks.

acute. Severe or sudden.

acute care facility. A hospital that provides care for patients requiring a stay for immediate attention and usually for a short period of time.

acute heart failure exacerbation. A worsening of the chronic condition in which the heart is not pumping blood efficiently.

acute myocardial infarction (AMI). Heart attack.

adrenal glands. The glands sitting on top of your kidney that are responsible for making steroids.

adrenal insufficiency. A condition in which the adrenal glands are not making steroids properly.

advanced. Describes the process of moving the patient along toward recovery and normalcy, for example, by a diet that changes from a liquid to a more regular consistency.

advanced care for elders (ACE) units. Areas using a specialized approach to prevent the decline elderly patients can have in the hospital.

advance directive. A document outlining what the patient wants done if something catastrophic occurs (heart or breathing stops, brain function is compromised).

adverse events. Unwanted and potential problems resulting from medical treatment.

ambulating. Walking.

ambulatory surgery centers (ASC) (surgicenters, same-day surgery centers). Outpatient surgery centers.

anemic. Possessing a low number of red blood cells, which are responsible for carrying oxygen throughout the body.

anesthesiologist. A doctor trained in using medication to induce sleep and to prevent pain during and after surgery.

angiogram. A test involving dye that shows the veins and arteries of the body.

angioplasty. A procedure that opens a blocked blood vessel.

ankle-brachia index (ABI) analysis. A test that compares the blood pressure in the ankle with the blood pressure in the arm.

anticoagulant. Blood-thinning medication.

arrhythmia. Irregular heart rhythm.

arterial blood gas (ABG). Blood samples from arteries to measure oxygen and carbon dioxide.

arterial lines (A-lines). Catheters placed in the artery rather than the vein.

arteries. The vessels that carry blood with oxygen from the heart to the organs and tissues in the body.

arthrocentesis. A procedure used to remove fluid from joints.

aspiratation. (1) inhaling food or drink; (2) drawing off fluid with a needle from the tissues and organs in the body.

atrial fibrillation. An irregular rhythm of the heart.

atrophy. Wasting or weakening.

attending of record. The physician who has ultimate responsibility for the patient's care.

attending physician (attending). The professional who completed medical education and residency and who has responsibility for the patient's care.

automatic implantable cardioverter-defibrillator (AICD). A device that senses the heart rhythm and can shock the heart out of a dangerous rhythm or administer a shock if the heart stops.

axillary vein. One of two vessels that convey blood from the armpit to the heart.

barium. A chemical substance that can be seen in an X-ray.

barium swallow. A test in which the patient drinks a liquid containing barium while X-rays are taken to determine the cause of a swallowing problem.

baseline. (1)The patient's condition before admission to the hospital; (2)the first version of a test, against which subsequent versions will be compared.

basic metabolic panel (chemistry). The test that looks at the levels of sodium, potassium, blood urea nitrogen (BUN), creatinine, and glucose in the blood.

bilirubin. A fluid made in the liver.

biocontainment unit. An extremely specialized unit to monitor patients and to protect others from contracting highly dangerous contagious infections such as Ebola and SARS.

biopsy. Removal of a piece of tissue or organ to examine in a laboratory to evaluate the presence of cancer or other disease.

bladder. The organ that collects the urine made by the kidneys.

blanching. Whitening of the skin after pressure is placed.

blood glucose. Sugar present in the blood.

blood test; blood work. A general term for many different types of tests performed on blood drawn from the patient.

blood urea nitrogen (BUN). In a blood test, a substance that indicates kidney function.

bolused. Delivered all at once, as with medication.

bone marrow biopsy. A test using a needle to draw off fluid from inside the bone, where the various blood cells are made; used to diagnose certain types of cancer.

bronchoscopy. A procedure in which a scope is inserted into the trachea (windpipe) and down into the bronchus (large airway in the lungs) to take pictures and tissue samples.

burn center. A unit with highly trained professionals and specialized equipment where patients with severe and life-threatening burns are treated. See also **hyperbaric chamber.**

capsule endoscopy. A procedure in which a pill-sized camera is swallowed to take pictures of the small bowel.

cardiac arrest. The condition in which the heart has stopped.

cardiac care unit (CCU). A unit in the hospital where patients who have severe cardiac problems are cared for.

cardiac catheterization. A process in which a thin tube is inserted into the blood vessels, allowing visualization of the blood flow through the coronary arteries; can also be used to open up any blockages.

cardiac catheterization lab (cath lab). The unit where there is equipment to visualize the blood vessels around the heart and unblock arteries when necessary.

cardiac electrophysiologist. A cardiologist who specializes in heart rhythms.

cardiac output. The measure of blood flow out of the heart to the rest of the body.

cardiologist. An internal medicine doctor who has completed fellowship training in heart issues.

cardiothoracic care unit (CTU). The unit where patients are cared for in the hospital after (or occasionally before) cardiothoracic surgery.

cardiothoracic surgeons. Surgeons trained to operate on the heart and lungs.

cardioversion. An electric shock to the heart.

carotids. Large arteries in the neck that supply blood to the brain.

case manager (discharge planner). The professional who evaluates all the medical and social information to help determine where the patient should go after leaving the hospital.

catheter. A thin tube that is inserted in the body for surgery or to treat a medical condition.

catheter-associated urinary tract infection (CAUTI). A common infection in hospitals that results from the insertion of a tube into the urethra.

CBC (complete blood count). A set of tests to measure the cellular components in the blood: hemoglobin, hematocrit, white blood cell count, and platelet count.

C. diff. (Clostridium difficile). Bacteria that cause serious and highly contagious diarrhea.

central line (central venous catheter, central venous line, central venous access catheter). A tube placed in one of the large veins in the neck, chest, or groin; it is also identified by the number of ports—e.g., single lumen, double lumen, etc.

central line-associated bloodstream infections (CLABSI). An infection in the blood caused by the presence of a central line.

central veins. Large veins in the neck, chest, or groin.

cerebral vascular accident (CVA). A stroke.

charge nurse. The nurse who is responsible for the all the personnel and processes on a hospital unit.

chemistry (basic metabolic panel). The test that looks at the levels of sodium, potassium, blood urea nitrogen (BUN), creatinine, and glucose in the blood.

chemotherapy. A type or combination of medication to treat cancer or other diseases.

chest tube. A small plastic tube that is placed through the side of the chest into the space around the lungs.

chest X-ray. A test using radiation to examine the vital organs in the chest cavity; a routine test for patients coming to the hospital, it can diagnose pneumonia, pulmonary embolism, and other lung conditions.

chief complaint. The medical problem that causes an individual to seek treatment.

child life advocate. A trained specialist who uses tools and strategies through art or play to help hospitalized children sort through feelings.

cholecystectomy. Surgical gallbladder removal.

cholesterol. A fat substance found in the tissues in the body, believed to promote heart disease.

chronic. Ongoing and for a long period.

clinical pharmacists. Professionals with advanced training in the science of medications; often participate in patient rounds to advise providers.

clinical research coordinator (research nurse). The individual who enrolls patients in a clinical trial, collects their medical information, and schedules visits.

Clostridium difficile (C. diff.). Bacteria that cause serious and highly contagious diarrhea.

coagulation profile. A test that indicates the thinness of blood and is important for patients on certain blood-thinning medications.

coagulopathy. A bleeding disorder in which the blood does not clot as well as it should.

codes. Alerts to the medical or surgical team best suited to manage the emergency; may be called over the hospital intercom.

cognitive testing. A set of questions to determine whether a patient is thinking clearly and to rule out dementia.

cohorted. Grouped together.

colitis. Infection or inflammation of the large bowel (colon).

colonoscopy. A procedure that uses a scope to see inside the large intestines, often as a standard screening test for colon cancer.

colorectal surgeons. Surgeons trained to operate on the intestines.

comfort measures. Measures taken when no further testing, workup, or treatment is wanted.

community. Where you live, if it is not in a skilled nursing facility; this becomes an important piece of information to help providers understand what potential germs may be causing a patient's illness.

community hospital. Local hospital that provides a variety of basic services; ideal for routine care.

comorbid conditions. Illnesses in addition to the ones for which a patient is admitted.

compression stockings (TEDS). Devices that can be worn on the legs to keep blood flowing when the patient is either in bed or not walking very much.

compromised. Indicating that the immune system is weak and unable to fight off infections.

computed tomography (CT) or computed axial tomography (CAT) scan. Imaging process using radiation to see inside organs and structures; well suited for bone injuries, lung and chest imaging, and cancer detection.

confusion assessment method (CAM). A set of questions that may be asked at the bedside to evaluate patients for delirium.

congestive heart failure (CHF). A chronic condition in which the heart does not pump blood adequately.

consult. The situation in which a specialized doctor is called by another provider to evaluate a patient with a suspected medical problem within the specialist's field.

contact precautions. The measures everyone who enters a patient's room must take, including wearing disposable gowns and gloves, to avoid contracting and spreading contagious illnesses.

continuous bladder irrigation. The process of clearing blood from the bladder by injecting water through a specialized urinary catheter with three channels.

contraindicated for. Not allowed.

coronary arteries. The blood vessels that supply blood to the heart.

coronary bypass surgery or coronary artery bypass graft (CABG). Surgery to clear blockages in the heart vessels.

cortisol. A steroid hormone made in the adrenal glands; it is known as the "stress hormone" because it regulates many body functions in response to stress.

cosyntropin test. A test that evaluates pituitary and adrenal gland function by measuring a hormone produced by the adrenal gland.

C reactive protein (CRP). Blood test to assess the level of inflammation in the body.

creatinine. The byproduct of muscle waste breakdown; in a blood test it indicates kidney function.

culture (of a hospital). How a hospital is organized and how it is run; will vary from hospital to hospital.

cystoscopy. A procedure in which a thin scope is inserted up the urethra and into the bladder.

debridement. Removal of dead tissue.

deep vein thrombosis (DVT). A blood clot in a limb.

defibrillator. A machine that can deliver an electric shock to the chest.

delirium. An altered state of consciousness that waxes and wanes, characterized by confusion and agitation.

dermatologic. Related to a skin condition.

detoxification. A protocol to administer medication to prevent the symptoms of withdrawal from drugs and alcohol.

dialysis. A process that either filters the blood (hemo) or filters the fluid in the abdominal cavity (peritoneal) to get rid of toxins and to balance electrolytes for failing kidneys.

discharge disposition. Determination of where patients go after the hospital stay, whether home or to rehab.

discharge planner (case manager). The professional who evaluates all the medical and social information to help determine where the patient should go after leaving the hospital.

diverticulitis. Inflammation of small pouches in the colon (large intestine).

doctor's orders. Refers to the instructions physicians. or in some instances, nurse practitioners or physician assistants. create to direct patient care.

Do not resuscitate orders (DNR). Instructions to providers indicating that a patient does not wish to have cardiopulmonary resuscitation in the event that the heart stops beating or he or she cannot breathe.

Doppler. An ultrasound test using waves that shows blood flow.

drain. A thin plastic tube that allows fluid to exit the body; common after surgery and procedures.

dressing. A sterile bandage.

dysphagia. Difficulty swallowing.

echocardiogram. Ultrasound of the heart.

elective surgery. Planned surgery.

electrocardiogram (EKG). A test of a person's heart rhythm, displaying waves to indicate the heart's electrical activity.

electrolytes. The chemicals (calcium, magnesium, potassium, sodium, phosphate, and chloride) in the body that regulate many essential life functions.

electronic medical record (EMR). A computerized record that collects and maintains all the information about a patient, replacing paper charts.

electrophysiology (EP) testing or study. A test in which electrode catheters are threaded up to the heart to record electrical signals; can ablate the area of the heart that is sending out bad signals.

emergent. Indicating an urgent, life-threatening situation.

empyema. A pocket of pus in the pleural space around the lungs.

endoscopic retrograde cholangiopancreatography (ERCP). A procedure using a flexible lighted scope and X-rays to visualize the ducts that drain the liver, pancreas, and gallbladder.

endoscopic ultrasound (EUS). A test that combines an endoscopy and ultrasound.

endoscopy. A procedure using a scope to examine inside a hollow organ. usually referring to the procedure to look into the esophagus and stomach.

endotracheal (ET) tube. A tube that is inserted down into the trachea when breathing is difficult or prior to surgery.

enteric. Relating to the intestines.

environmental worker. Janitor.

error of commission. An error that occurs when something specifically incorrect was done or given to a patient.

error of omission. An error that occurs when the patient did not get the medication or procedure or provision of care necessary or the medication, procedure, or provision of care varied from what the medical profession calls the standard of care.

esophagogastroduodenoscopy (EGD). A procedure in which a scope is placed in the throat to visualize the esophagus, stomach, and first part of the small intestine.

esophagus. Food pipe.

ethics committee. A group of hospital members and/or lawyers who meet to help families, patients, and the health care professionals resolve moral and ethical dilemmas.

exercise stress test. A test in which an EKG (electrocardiogram) is administered while you are exercising to determine how much activity the heart can tolerate.

external jugular (EJ) venous catheter. A line placed in the peripheral vein in the neck.

fellow. A physician who has completed residency training and is getting extra years of training in a specialty (referred to as a fellowship).

femoral vein. A large vein in the groin.

fetal demise. Still birth or death of the fetus prior to delivery.

flora. In the body, this refers to bacteria.

fluoroscopy. A specialized continuous X-ray.

Foley catheter(urinary catheter). Flexible tubing that is placed into the bladder to collect urine.

Food and Drug Administration (FDA). The government agency that oversees the safety of foods and medications, including testing of new drugs.

formulary. Hospital pharmacy; oversees a set of medications that have the same properties as those of equivalent drugs.

free water. Fluids without particles. for example, water, carbonated drinks, coffee, and tea.

gastroenterologist. A physician specializing in stomach, liver, or intestine issues.

generalist. A primary care physician who takes care of a variety of medical issues.

GI (stress ulcer) prophylaxis. A preventive strategy in which hospitalized patients are given stomach acid-lowering medications to reduce the risk of stomach bleeding.

give report. In the nursing profession, to relay information about patients.

glucose. Blood sugar.

goals of care. A discussion with patients and families usually during a time of severe illness to make a plan of care based on the patient's and family's overall goals regarding the patients future quality of life.

gynecologic. Pertaining to female reproductive organs.

health care proxy. An individual entrusted to make medical decisions for another individual.

health system (health care system). A group of hospitals and health care facilities that is owned and managed centrally; may include rehabilitation centers, outpatient offices, and nursing homes.

hematocrit. A test that reveals the volume of the red blood cells that carry oxygen throughout the body.

hemodynamics. The flow of blood through the circulatory system.

hemoglobin. The protein in the blood that carries oxygen throughout the body.

hemoglobin A1C. A blood test to measure the level of glucose control over the previous three months.

heparin. A blood-thinning medication.

hold. To discontinue a medication, at least temporarily

homeostatic. Describes the body's natural tendency to keep all the functions and processes in balance.

hormones. Chemical substances that control functions and activities in the body.

hospice. A service that allows a patient to be palliated (cared for with comfort measures) in a facility such as a hospital, nursing home, or at home at the end of life.

hospitalists. Physicians who work only in the hospital and do not usually take care of patients on the outside.

hyperbaric chamber. An equipped space to treat certain conditions with oxygen therapy, it is part of a specialized burn unit.

hyperthyroidism. Overactivity of the thyroid gland; associated with rapid metabolism.

hypothyroidism. Underactivity of the thyroid gland; associated with slow metabolism.

imaging. Tests that obtain pictures.

immunocompromised. Identifies patients whose bodies are unable to fend off infection.

implants. An artificial device inserted into the body.

incision and drainage. Surgical cut to allow fluid to exit the body.

indication. The medical reason for doing something.

induce. To begin or start a process; may refer to anesthesia or childbirth labor.

infective endocarditis. Inflammation of the inner tissue of the heart, typically by bacteria.

influenza (flu). A virus spread through the air by droplets; it is highly contagious and can be dangerous for certain classes of individuals (elderly, immunocompromised).

INR. A blood test that reveals how thin the blood is by timing how long it takes to clot.

insulin. The substance made by the pancreas to enable the body to use sugar; patients with diabetes take insulin medication to control sugars.

intensive care unit (ICU). A specialized part of the hospital for patients who need extra attention; also referred to as critical care and special care unit.

intensivist. The physician specialist who supervises care of patients in an ICU.

interdisciplinary rounds. An organized hospital process in which different specialties and professionals come together to discuss patients' conditions, treatments, and outlook; may occur at the bedside or outside the patient's room.

intermediate care unit (step-down unit). An area for patients judged not sick enough for the ICU but who need more medical attention than the regular floor can provide.

intern. A physician in the first year of residency; it can also refer to other health care professionals in training.

internal bleeds. Bleeding that is not visible.

internal jugular. A large vein in the neck.

interventional cardiologist. A physician trained in using procedures to treat heart conditions.

interventional radiologist. A physician trained in using imaging to perform treatment procedures.

intravenous line (IV). A small plastic tubing that is placed in a peripheral vein.

intra-aortic balloon pump (IABP). A machine used to help increase the output of the heart.

intubated. Having an endotracheal tube for mechanical ventilation (machine-assisted breathing).

invasive. Describes a test or procedure that enters through the skin or into a body cavity.

isolation. A measure to either protect patients against infection or prevent others from being exposed to a highly contagious illness.

Jackson-Pratt (JP) drain. A drainage device that works on a suction mechanism.

jejunum. The second part of the small intestine.

jejunostomy tube (J tube). A tube that is passed from the stomach into the jejunum.

joint arthroplasty. Joint (knees, hips, shoulders) replacement surgery.

joint aspiration. Drawing fluid from a joint space.

laparoscopic surgery. An operation performed by the creation of tiny holes through which instruments are inserted into the abdomen and then controlled by the surgeon.

lidocaine. A numbing anesthetic to decrease pain.

lines. Tubes, sometimes known as catheters, that can be placed in arteries or veins and can be located peripherally or centrally.

liquid tumors. Cancers that affect the bone marrow and are usually either lymphoma or leukemia.

lithotripsy. A procedure in which shock waves are directed at kidney stones to break them up so they can be passed in the urine.

living will. A document stating the patient's wishes for the extent and limits of treatment.

lumbar puncture (spinal tap). A procedure in which a needle is inserted into the spinal canal to extract cerebrospinal fluid for analysis.

lumen. (1) In a catheter, describes the component tubes; (2) in the body, describes the inside of a tubular structure such as an artery or vein.

magnetic resonance imaging (MRI). A test using magnetic energy waves that gives different information about the structures inside the body than X-ray and CT scans do; not safe for individuals with metal implants.

managing. In medicine, taking care of a patient's medical needs and treatment.

mapping. In radiation therapy, a process to determine where the beams will be directed and how many treatments of radiation are needed.

mechanical obstruction. Blockage.

medical center. A health care facility or group of hospitals with many different types of services.

medical intensive care unit (MICU). A unit in a hospital in which adult patients with severe general medical issues are taken care of and may receive extra attention and monitoring.

medical optimization. Ensuring that patients, and particularly their heart and lungs, are in the best possible condition before going under anesthesia.

medication reconciliation (medrec). A review of medications at admission and discharge.

medicine service. The general name for primary care and specialties concerned with internal medicine.

med-surg unit. A unit in the hospital in which both medical and surgical patients are placed.

metabolic equivalents (METS). How energy is measured in the body; the unit is calories.

metabolism. All the chemical and physical processes that sustain the body.

midlevel provider. A term used to refer to nurse practitioners and physician assistants.

midline. A line that falls in between a regular peripheral IV and a PICC line. It is longer than a regular peripheral IV but does not pass the axillary line (in the armpit).

mini mental status exam (MMSE). A thirty-point questionnaire to assess orientation and specific cognitive skills used to diagnose dementia.

monitor. (1) Equipment that measures the body's functions electronically; (2) to keep watch over a patient when there is cause for concern.

MRSA (methicillin-resistant Staphylococcus aureus). A kind of staph bacterium that does not respond to antibiotics, often referred to as the super bug.

MVA. Motor vehicle accident.

nasal cannula. Plastic tubing that rests in the nostrils and delivers oxygen.

nasogastric (NGT or NG) tube. A flexible plastic tube placed down the nose through the esophagus and into the stomach for feeding.

negative pressure isolation. The situation in which a patient is put in a negative pressure room to prevent transmission of disease from the patient to others.

negative pressure room. A room that allows air to enter but not exit as a wayto decrease the spread of illnesses.

neonatal intensive care unit (NICU). The unit in the hospital where newborn and premature babies are taken when they need extra care.

neonates. Newborn babies.

nephrologist. A physician specializing in kidney issues.

nephrostomy tube. A small plastic tube that passes from the skin to a part of the patient's kidney. Bags are attached to the tubes to collect the urine.

neurologist. A physician who specializes in the nervous system.

neurosurgeons. Surgeons trained to operate on the brain and spine.

neurosurgical care unit (NSCU). A unit in the hospital where adult patients with severe brain or spinal cord injuries are taken care of.

neutropenic fever. A fever in a patient with a low white blood cell count.

nontunneled catheter. A fixed line that protrudes at the site of an insertion and does not dwell under the skin.

NPO. Abbreviation for the Latin phrase *non per os,* meaning nothing by mouth, referring to no food or drink.

nuclear stress test. A test in which a radioactive tracer is injected into a vein to evaluate blood flow to the heart.

NSAIDs (nonsteriodal antiflammatory drugs). Nonnarcotic, nonsteroidal pain medications, such as aspirin, ibuprofen, and naproxen sodium.

nurse's aide. The paraprofessional who works with the RN to take care of basic patient needs such as bathing, feeding, and toileting.

nurse burnout. The physical, emotional, and psychological stress that RNs are subject to as a consequence of excess burdens in rendering patient care.

nurse manager. The RN professional who has responsibility for the all the personnel and processes on a particular unit or service.

nurse practitioner (NP). An advanced practice nurse with graduate training; can assume primary care responsibilities.

obstetrical. Referring to maternity.

occluded. Blocked.

off service and *on service.* Describing when a physician is or is not covering an inpatient team of patients.

Ommaya reservoir. A type of port for chemotherapy to the brain.

oncologist. A doctor specializing in cancer.

optimization. The process of healthful preparation before surgery or a procedure.

OR. Operating room.

orderlies (or transporters). Hospital staff members who bring patients from one area to another, typically on stretchers or on wheelchairs.

orthopaedic surgeons. Doctors specializing in bone and cartilage issues.

otolaryngologists (ENTs). Surgeons trained to operate on ear, nose, and throat.

oxygen (O_2). The primary gas component in the air we breathe; may be given supplementally to help breathing.

palliate. Care for with comfort measures.

palliative care. A set of principles focused on end-of-life comforts.

paracentesis. A procedure to remove fluid from the abdomen.

pathogens. Disease-causing germs.

pathologist. The physician specialist who examines cells and tissue at the microscopic level to look for disease.

patient-care associate or assistant (PCA). Nurse's aide.

patient controlled analgesic (PCA) pump. An intravenous line that delivers pain medication and is placed in a peripheral vein.

patient handoff. One health care professional communicating all the information relative to the patient's care to another health care professional.

pediatric intensive care unit (PICU). The unit in the hospital where infants through adolescents are taken care of for advanced or serious medical illnesses or injuries.

pelvic exam. An internal examination of the structures in the female reproductive system.

pelvic ultrasound. A noninvasive procedure, performed with an ultrasound probe over the abdomen or an additional probe placed in the vagina for a female and the rectum for a male.

percutaneous gastrostomy tube (PEG or feeding tube). A tube placed into the stomach that delivers nutrition.

perfusion. Blood flow.

peribottle. A bottle used after delivery of a baby to spray the bottom with warm water in place of toilet paper.

perioperative period. The time right before and for a short time after surgery.

peripheral arterial disease (PAD). Narrowing of the arteries.

peripherally inserted central catheter (PICC line). An intravenous line that can remain in the body for thirty days.

peripheral vein. A vein in the arms, legs, hands, or feet.

permanent pacemaker (PPM). A device that regulates heart rate.

phlebotomists. Technicians who have had special training to draw patient blood.

physician assistant (PA). A health care professional who has undergone years of classroom and practical training to practice medicine or surgery under the supervision of a physician.

physician extenders. A term previously used to refer to nurse practitioners and physician assistants.

physical therapists (PTs). The professionals trained to help patients move and regain mobility.

placebeo. A fake or dummy drug, used for testing in clinical trials.

placed. Inserted.

platelets. The blood cells that promote the clotting process.

platelet count. A measurement of the blood component that informs how well the blood clots.

pleura. A tissue that covers the lungs and inside of the ribs.

pleural effusion. A collection of fluid in the pleural space.

pleural space. A small space between the two layers of tissues that surround the lungs.

pneumothorax. A condition in which air gets into the pleural space and the lung collapses.

port (Medi-Port, Port-a-Cath, Infuse-a-Port). A tunneled catheter that is left completely under the skin.

post-anesthesia care unit (PACU, recovery room). The unit to which patients go right after surgery while they are still waking up from the anesthesia.

postoperative ileus. Slowing down of the bowel after surgery or procedures.

post-void residual sonography. An ultrasound over the bladder after the bladder has been emptied.

potassium. An electrolyte important for proper cardiac function.

pressors. A class of medications to increase blood pressure.

pressure ulcers (bedsores). Irritations in and through the skin that occur when patients are unable to move; they can be serious and a cause of infection.

presurgical testing. The collection of information through physical examination, bloodwork, imaging, and history taking to ensure that a patient can safely undergo surgery.

primary care provider (PCP). A medical health care professional involved in the overall care of a patient.

privileges. Permission given to physicians to admit and treat patients at a specific hospital.

prophylaxis. Prevention.

prosthetic. Artificial.

protocol. A set of rules or guidelines designed to help medical professionals and staff take care of patients in a standardized, uniform way.

PTT. Blood test that reveals how thin your blood is by timing how long it takes the blood to clot.

pulmonary artery. The large blood vessel connecting the right ventricle of the heart to the lungs.

pulmonary embolism (PE). A blood clot that has traveled to a vessel in the lung.

pulmonary function tests. Breathing tests.

pulmonologist. A physician specializing in lung issues.

pulse oximetry. A measurement taken noninvasively on the finger to see if blood is getting enough oxygen.

radiation therapy. The use of radiation for treatment as opposed to diagnosis.

radiograph. The official name for an X-ray, an imaging technique that uses radiation to visualize structures inside the body.

radiographic studies. A series of images.

radiology technician (tech). An individual with training to administer any of the imaging forms.

radiotracer. A chemical substance that is injected that allows pictures of inside the body.

rapid sequence induction. The process of getting the patient under anesthesia and beginning the operation as quickly as possible.

recovered. After surgery, returned to the best possible state of breathing and alertness under the watchful care of specialized staff.

rectal tube. A tube that is placed in the rectum to relieve diarrhea or gas.

refer. Term used when a physician sends the patient to a specialist or higher-level hospital for specific care or a specialized procedure.

registered dietitian (RD). A professional who has had education and training about human physiology and nutrition science.

registered nurse (RN). A professional with education and training in patient care who has passed a licensing exam.

registration. The process in which information about name, address, next of kin, and insurance is collected upon arrival at the hospital.

rehabilitation facility (rehab). A center where patients who require ongoing therapy outside a hospital receive care.

relationship-based care. The practice of including patients and families in care decisions.

resident (house staff, house officer). Physician trainee who has graduated from medical school; they perform the same duties as senior physicians but under their supervision.

residue. Dietary fiber.

respirator(ventilator). Breathing machine for patients who cannot breathe on their own.

respiratory therapist (RT). Individual trained to take care of patients with lung problems.

resuscitate. The act of reviving a patient who has stopped breathing or whose heart has stopped beating.

reverse isolation. Measures to prevent patients from acquiring illness brought by staff or visitors.

risk stratification. A process to predict how groups of patients will recover or survive, which takes into account a set of factors.

rotations. Residency training through different hospitals for exposure to various types and environments of medical care.

rounds. (1)The time when providers officially see patients in the hospital; (2) "to round": the act by providers of examining, diagnosing, and treating patients.

ruling out. The process to determine that a patient does not have a suspected specific illness or problem.

same-day admit. A patient's admission to the hospital without spending the night before surgery there.

scalpel. Surgical knife.

secondary to. In medicine, as a result of.

secondary care hospital. A hospital with an intermediate level of care between that provided by a community hospital and that of a tertiary care hospital.

sedation vacation. A patient's removal from sleep-inducing medication for a short time.

sedimentation rate. A blood test that assesses the level of inflammation in the body.

semi-emergent. In medicine, referring to a condition warranting attention in the near term but not quite an emergency.

sepsis. An overwhelming infection.

sequential compression devices. Devices that surround the legs and periodically compress them to keep the blow flowing well.

service. Refers to the main specialty in charge of the patient's care—e.g., neurology, medicine, or surgery.

short-stay units. Units for patients who need to be monitored, treated briefly, or stabilized before being discharged

skilled nursing facility/nursing home (SNF). A health care institution for patients who are either temporarily or permanently unable to care for themselves.

skin biopsy. A small sample of skin taken surgically to evaluate it for cancer or other diseases.

social supports. Network of family and friends.

social worker. A professional with training to help people adjust and cope with adverse conditions.

sodium. The medical term for the chemical salt.

sodium level. How much salt is present in the circulating blood.

solarium. In previous eras, a room or large porch where patients were exposed to sunlight.

solid tumors. Cancers of the organs such as brain, breast, lung, pancreas, and colon.

specialist. An internist physician who has had advanced training in a specific area.

standard of care. The agreed-upon best way to treat a disorder or perform a medical procedure.

stenosis. The constriction or narrowing of any opening in the body.

stent. A tiny tube to hold an artery open to allow easy blood flow.

step-down unit (intermediate care unit). An area for patients judged not sick enough for the ICU but who need more medical attention than the regular floor can provide.

Stevens Johnson syndrome. Severe blistering of the skin's top layer, typically brought on by a drug reaction.

stress echocardiography. A test in which an echocardiogram is used to evaluate blood flow to the heart.

stress test. A test that assesses the blood flow to the heart while it is being challenged by strenuous exercise or medication.

study. In medicine, a test.

subacute facility. A rehabilitation center or skilled nursing facility that provides care and supervision for patients not well enough to return home after hospital discharge.

subclavian vein. A large vein in the chest.

sundowning. Confusion of a patient in the evening.

superior vena cava. The large vein that brings blood back to the heart.

superspecialist. A physician with training in and focus on a highly specific area of medicine.

surgical intensive care unit (SICU). The ICU where patients with surgical complications or possibly very complex, long surgeries are taken care of so that they can receive extra attention and monitoring.

surgical wound. The site where the incision was made.

sutured. Sewn into the skin to hold it in place.

Swan-Ganz (pulmonary artery) catheter. A catheter placed in the pulmonary artery through a central line.

syncope. Fainting or passing out.

teaching hospital. A hospital that incorporates residents, medical students, student nurses, and other health care professionals into patient care processes under supervision.

tele-ICU, eICU, electronic ICU. The use of audiovisual monitoring, computers, and telephones to perform health care from a remote location.

telemetry monitoring. Continuous heart monitoring, often implemented for heart-related complaints such as chest pain or syncope.

terminal clean. A process using specific protocols and products to kill and prevent the spread of communicable diseases.

tertiary care hospital. A hospital that offers a variety of highly specialized services and equipment beyond general medical, surgical, and obstetrical care.

therapeutic interchange. The substitution of one medication for another equivalent or similar medication.

therapeutic value. The ability of a medication to be effective.

thoracentesis. A procedure to remove fluid from the space around the lungs.

thorascopic surgery. An operation by the creation of tiny holes through which instruments are inserted into the chest and then controlled by the surgeon.

thyroid scan. A test using radioactivity to take pictures to examine activity in the thyroid gland.

tilt table. A diagnostic test to determine the cause of dizziness or passing out.

total parenteral nutrition (TPN) or *parenteral nutrition (PN).* A form of feeding that bypasses the gastrointestinal system.

TPA. A clot-busting medication.

trachea. Windpipe, the tube by which air is taken into the lungs.

tracheostomy. A hole cut in the trachea (windpipe) through which a plastic breathing tube is inserted and connected to a ventilator (breathing machine).

transesophageal echo (TEE). An echocardiogram in which a scope is placed down the throat into the esophagus to get a better look at part of the back of the heart.

transaminases. Liver enzymes.

transfer. In a medical context, to transport a patient from one health care facility to another.

transfusion. The process of putting blood or blood products into the body.

transthoracic echo (TTE). An echocardiogram that allows visualization of the structure of the heart and the blood flow across these structures.

triage. An emergency department process of evaluating new patients to determine how serious their medical situation is and how quickly they must be seen by a medical provider.

triage nurse. A nurse in the emergency department who evaluates incoming patients.

triglycerides. Substance that reveals the level of fat in the blood.

tunneled catheter. Line inserted at one site, tunneled under the skin, emerging at a separate site.

twenty-four-hour urine testing. A test in which urine is collected over a twenty-four-hour period for analysis at a laboratory, used to determine protein levels.

type and screen. A blood test to determine the blood type and factors.

ultrasound. An imaging method using sound waves to visualize inside the body.

underlying conditions. Existing medical illnesses.

unit clerk or *unit secretary.* A person who coordinates the flow of patients, transporters, reports, charts, personnel, and all information on a unit.

university hospital or medical center. A facility that is integrally associated with a medical school; there is likely to be active research, and many of the physicians are professors involved in teaching.

unstable arrhythmia. Abnormal rhythm of the heart.

unstable condition. One in which the patient is very ill and at risk.

ureter. The structure that carries urine from the kidney to the bladder.

urethra. The structure that carries urine out of the body from the bladder.

urinary catheter (Foley catheter). Flexible tubing that is placed into the bladder to collect urine.

veins. The vessels that return blood to the heart and lungs to pick up more oxygen.

venipuncture. Drawing blood through a vein; involves piercing the skin.

Venodyne (sequential compression device). A device that surrounds and periodically compresses the legs to stimulate blood flow.

venous thromboembolism. A blood clot that originates from a vein.

ventilation/perfusion (V/Q) scan. A procedure in which the patient inhales an aerosolized radioactive material through a mouthpiece and is scanned by a camera to compare blood flow and air movement.

ventilator (respirator). A machine that breathes for the patient who is unable to breathe independently.

video-assisted thorascopic surgery (VATS). Surgery to get into the lungs with a small camera to perform biopsies and procedures.

vital signs. A set of closely monitored medical parameters that give health care providers information about a patient's medical status.

vitamin K antagonist. A substance that prevents the proper functioning of certain blood-clotting factors.

void. To empty the bladder.

warfarin (Coumadin). A blood-thinning (anticoagulant) medication.

weaning. The process of decreasing an individual's dependence on something to which he or she has become accustomed; in the hospital environment, may refer to gradually taking a patient off mechanical ventilation.

white blood cell count. A measure of the components of the blood that fight off infections.

workup. A detective-like process of figuring out what is troubling a patient; may include history taking, physical exam, blood and urine samples, medication review, and imaging.

X-ray. An imaging technique that uses radiation to visualize structures inside the body.

INDEX